the

CBD OIL SOLUTION

the

CBD OIL
SOLUTION

Treat chronic pain, anxiety, insomnia, and more—without the high

DR. RACHNA PATEL

Recipes by Sandra Hinchliffe

ALPHA

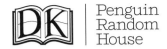

Publisher Mike Sanders
Editor Ann Barton
Book Designer Lindsay Dobbs
Art Director William Thomas
Recipe Developer Sandra Hinchliffe
Photography Eric Lubrick
Food Styling Savannah Norris
Proofreader Monica Stone
Indexer Celia McCoy

First American Edition, 2019
Published in the United States by DK Publishing
6081 E. 82nd Street, Indianapolis, Indiana 46250

Text, excluding recipes, copyright © 2019 Rachna Patel
Recipes copyright © 2019 Dorling Kindersley Limited
A Penguin Random House company
19 20 21 22 23 10 9 8 7 6 5 4
005–312955–MAR2019

Published in the United States by Dorling Kindersley Limited

ISBN: 978-1-4654-8076-7
Library of Congress Catalog Number: 2018958036

DK books are available at special discounts when purchased in bulk for sales promotions, premiums, fund-raising, or educational use. For details, contact: DK Publishing Special Markets, 1450 Brodway, Suite 801, New York, NY 10018 or SpecialSales@dk.com.

Printed and bound in Latvia

A WORLD OF IDEAS:
SEE ALL THERE IS TO KNOW

www.dk.com

To the most amazing human being I know,
whom I'm lucky enough to call my dad.

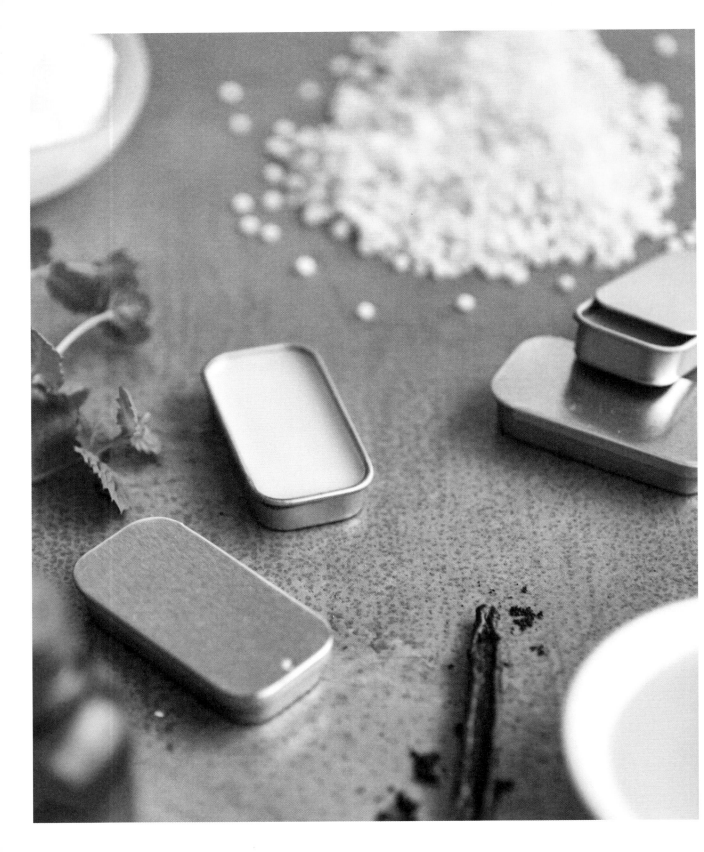

CONTENTS

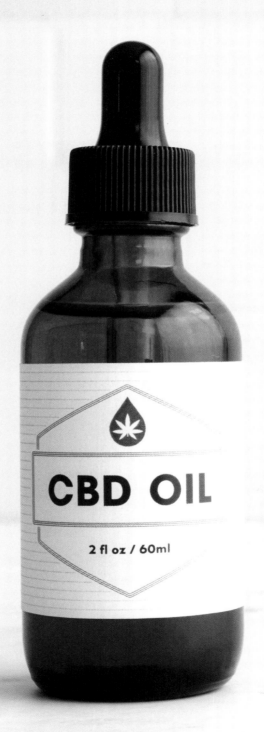

INTRODUCTION

Hey, there! I wanted to take a minute to personally introduce you to this book.

In all likelihood, you're struggling. You're looking for a solution to your problem—whether it's chronic pain, anxiety, insomnia, or some other medical condition. You've tried conventional medications, and they just aren't working. Maybe you've even considered using medical marijuana, but you're worried about the high.

You picked up this book in hopes of experiencing the benefits of marijuana without the high—by using CBD oil. You, my friend, picked up just the right book. Here you'll find everything you need to know about CBD oil, from what it is, to how to buy it and use it safely, as well as a selection of recipes for incorporating CBD oil into your everyday life.

As a physician, I've helped countless people just like you, who are struggling with chronic medical conditions. I've had patients completely eliminate their prescription medications and just use CBD oil to manage their symptoms. The effects of CBD oil have rippled into other parts of their lives—from work to relationships to leisure time. When symptoms are better managed, it leads to a better quality of life. And a better quality of life translates to more love, more laughter, and more happiness.

Hearing about these results touches my soul. I hope you find the information I have to share just as helpful as my patients have. I'm truly honored that you picked up this book, and I look forward to helping you.

With gratitude,

Rachna Patel

Dr. Rachna Patel

PART 1:
WHAT IS CBD OIL?

CBD, short for *cannabidiol,* is one of the many chemicals found in cannabis. Unlike tetrhydrocannbinol (THC), the other notorious and notable chemical compound found in cannabis, CBD does not have a psychoactive effect. In other words, it doesn't get you high, but it does effectively relieve a wide range of medical conditions, including chronic pain, anxiety, insomnia, and more.

One of the most commonly available and easily accessible forms of CBD is CBD oil. CBD oil is a concentrated extract from the cannabis family of plants that contains much higher amounts of CBD than THC.

Although CBD oil and other products made with CBD are becoming more popular and widespread, there are still a lot of misconceptions and misinformation about what CBD is and how it should be used. In this section, we'll look at what CBD oil is, where it comes from, and how it's made.

WHERE DOES CBD COME FROM?

Cannabidoil (CBD) is one of hundreds of chemicals found in the cannabis family of plants. Plants in the cannabis family have been divided into two categories: hemp, sometimes called *industrial hemp,* and marijuana, often just called *cannabis.* While hemp and marijuana plants are part of the same family and share many commonalities, they differ when it comes to cultivation and use.

Hemp is used to make paper, clothing, and food, like protein powder and milk. It's also the main source of CBD used to make CBD oil and other CBD products. Marijuana is primarily grown for medical and recreational purposes and can also be used to make CBD oil.

The single greatest difference between hemp and marijuana is a legal one. It boils down to the amount of THC in the plant. Hemp has less than 0.3 percent THC; marijuana, by default, has more than 0.3 percent THC.

> **CBD (cannabidoil)** and **THC (tetrahydrocannabinol)** are two of the many chemical compounds, or cannabinoids, produced by the cannabis plant.

Why 0.3 percent? Way back when, a Canadian named Ernest Small arbitrarily decided to define hemp as having less than 0.3 percent THC, and it's stuck around since. In fact, it's become an internationally accepted standard.

Of the CBD oil products available on the market today, the vast majority of them are made with hemp. The ones that are made with marijuana are typically available through medical marijuana dispensaries.

So, long story short, CBD is present in all cannabis plants, both marijuana and hemp. However, most CBD products are made from hemp-derived CBD.

Cannabis

Hemp	Marijuana
• Lower THC (<0.3%) • Cultivated for a wide variety of uses, including textiles, plastics, food products, and biofuels.	• Higher THC (>0.3%, usually 5–30%) • Cultivated for medical and recreational use.

CBD from Hemp vs. CBD from Marijuana

You may be wondering, is there a difference between the CBD that comes from hemp and the CBD comes from marijuana? The answer is that CBD itself is CBD, whether it comes from hemp or from marijuana. In other words, the CBD from hemp has the same molecular structure as CBD from marijuana. Your body's not going to know the difference between the two.

However, there is a difference between the CBD oil (or other products) derived from hemp and the CBD oil derived from marijuana. The hemp-derived oil has less THC in it (below 0.3 percent), and the marijuana-derived CBD oil (sometimes called cannabis-derived oil) has more THC in it.

Depending on the medical condition being treated, the presence of THC can be an advantage or a disadvantage. The general perception out there is that the totality of the medical benefits are derived soley from CBD, but, in fact, that's not the case. While it's true that some medical conditions do benefit more from CBD, there are other conditions that benefit more from THC. And then there are medical conditions that benefit from both THC and CBD. See Part 4 for more about which chemical compound most benefits specific medical conditions.

A CLOSER LOOK AT CBD AND THC

As we've learned, cannabis plants produce many different cannabinoids, or chemical compounds, including CBD and THC. These are distinctly different compounds with different effects on the body.

The molecular structure of THC

The molecular structure of CBD

When consumed, both CBD and THC interact with receptors in the endocannabinoid system. This is a system that plays a regulatory role in a wide range of physiological and cognitive functions, including pain modulation, mood, and seizure threshold. You can think of the endocannabinoid system as a collection of locks and keys. The locks are located on cells, with many different keys floating around. The keys may be either endogenously produced (created by our bodies) or added exogenously (such as by taking a medication).

CBD and THC are both exogenously introduced "keys" that interact differently with the cannabinoid receptors ("locks") in the endocannabinoid system, so they have significantly different effects on the body. Unlike CBD, THC is psychoactive, which means it causes a high.

Why Does THC Get You High?

In simple terms, THC attaches itself to cannabinoid receptor 1 (CB-1) in the brain. Like a key in a lock, THC snuggly fits right into CB-1, and as a result of this interaction, the brain releases dopamine. The release of dopamine, in turn, affects things like mood, cognition, and perception. The total sum of all these changes creates that feeling that we've come to call a *high*.

If you smoked pot in your friend's basement back in high school, now you know why you scarfed down the entire party pack from Taco Bell, why your heart felt like it was racing, and why you found yourself crouching under the table, paranoid about an alien invasion. That, my friend, was the high caused by THC.

However, the mere presence of THC doesn't automatically lead to paranoia and insatiable munchies. It's important to know that these psychoactive effects generally kick in only after consuming way too much THC. The psychoactive effects of THC can typically be avoided when it is used at the right dose. Your doctor can help you find the dose that's right for you so that you don't get high from the THC.

Why Doesn't CBD Get You High?

Unlike THC, CBD doesn't fit snuggly into CB-1. Instead, it changes the shape of CB-1 in such a way that THC can't attach to it. Because of this, mood, cognition, and perception aren't affected, and there's no feeling of that high.

While preventing THC from causing a high, CBD interacts with a myriad of other target receptors throughout the body, unlocking a series of chemical reactions that lead to effects like pain relief, a calm and relaxed feeling, restful sleep, and more.

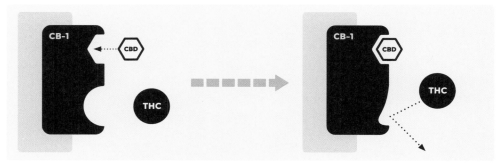

CBD acts as a negative allosteric inhibitor, changing the shape of CB-1 and preventing THC from attaching to this receptor.

HOW IS CBD OIL MADE?

CBD oil in its most basic form is made of two components, an extract and a carrier. The extract consists of the chemical compounds withdrawn from the hemp plant, which are typically then concentrated. The chemical compounds can be extracted using carbon dioxide, ethanol, hydrocarbon, or an oil. The other component is a carrier, which is typically an oil. A carrier oil is utilized to make the CBD extract more suitable for consumption.

Supercritical Carbon Dioxide Extraction

At room temperature and standard atmospheric pressure, carbon dioxide (CO_2) is a gas, but at cooler temperatures and higher pressures, it turns into a liquid. To extract CBD, liquid carbon dioxide saturates the hemp plant material and drips through. As soon as the temperature warms up and the pressure drops, the carbon dioxide reverts back to a gas and evaporates, leaving behind a highly concentrated CBD extract. To make CBD oil, the extract is then mixed with a carrier or base. CO_2 extraction is considered relatively non-toxic and is the preferred method of extraction in the hemp industry.

Ethanol Extraction

You may not be familiar with the word *ethanol,* but does the word *alcohol* ring a bell? Yup, that's right—alcohol, otherwise known as *ethanol,* is used to make CBD oil. In this process, ethanol is poured over the hemp plant material. The hemp is allowed to sit in the ethanol for several hours or up to a couple days. Then the mixture is filtered, leaving behind ethanol saturated with CBD. Next, the CBD-saturated ethanol is heated to evaporate the ethanol, leaving behind a highly concentrated CBD extract, which can then be mixed with a carrier or base to create CBD oil.

Ethanol is generally regarded as safe (GRAS) by the US Food and Drug Administration (FDA) and is an active ingredient in some hand sanitizers and medical wipes. That's because it's effective in killing most bacteria, fungi, and many viruses—an important factor to consider for those with compromised immune systems. The trade-off is that ethanol also coextracts chlorophyll, which means an ethanol-based CBD oil might taste like fresh grass clippings.

Hydrocarbon Extraction

A hydrocarbon is a chemical made of up hydrogen and carbon. The most common hydrocarbons used to extract CBD from hemp are butane, propane, hexane, and naphtha. In this process, the hydrocarbon is passed through the hemp plant material, which draws out the CBD. The residual solvent is then removed using heat and a vacuum. The heat evaporates the hydrocarbon and the vacuum suctions away the hydrocarbon evaporate (a process known as a *purge* or *purging*), leaving behind a highly concentrated CBD extract. The remaining extract can then be mixed with a carrier oil or base to create CBD oil.

Not every CBD extract goes through a purge, and improper purging leaves behind traces of the hydrocarbon. Even if the purging is done properly, it can be difficult to completely purge 100 percent of these hydrocarbons from the hemp extracts. The possibility of trace hydrocarbons, which pose health risks, makes this form of extraction less desirable than CO_2 or ethanol extraction.

Oil Extraction

Oil extraction uses an oil to extract the CBD. Olive oil, grapeseed oil, and medium-chain triglyceride (MCT) oil are the most common oils used to make CBD oil. (MCT oil is made by extracting and isolating medium-chain triglycerides from coconut oil. In general, MCT oil has no taste or smell.)

To extract the CBD in an oil itself, a glass container filled with hemp plant material and an oil is placed over a pan of boiling water—a double boiler, essentially—and heated. Once the mixture cools, it's filtered and the CBD oil is ready for consumption.

The trade-off to oil extraction is that these oils cannot be further concentrated, meaning patients may need to consume more in order to get the same medical benefits as from a CBD oil made using one of the other extraction methods.

CBD IN THE PAST...

The medical use of the cannabis plant dates back to ancient times. Around the world—from China to India to Egypt—it's been used for insomnia, headaches, gastrointestinal disorders, labor pain, menstrual pain, nerve pain, and more.

In the United States, cannabis was widely available in over-the-counter remedies until 1937. It fact, it was listed in the United States Pharmacopeia (USP) way back in 1850, only to be dropped in 1942. But, a mere half century later, it resurfaced again when California became the first state to legalize the medical use of cannabis in 1996, picking up where history left off.

Today, US laws are leaning more and more in favor of the medical use of cannabis, and we're once again witnessing the medical potential of the chemicals derived from cannabis, especially CBD.

In 2018, the FDA for the first time approved a pharmaceutical drug that contains a cannabinoid—CBD—derived from cannabis. This pharmaceutical drug goes by the trade name Epidiolex, and the generic name is—yup, you guessed it—*cannabidiol* (CBD). It's an oral solution approved for the treatment of seizures associated with two rare and severe forms of epilepsy, Lennox-Gastaut syndrome and Dravet syndrome.

The approval of Epidiolex marks an important step forward in medicine. It legitimizes CBD within the medical community, while also paving the way for more research related to cannabinoids.

...AND FOR THE FUTURE

As the benefits of CBD and other cannabinoids become increasingly recognized and studied, there's hope for their role in mitigating the current opioid crisis in the United States. Opioids, such as Norco, Percocet, and morphine, are a class of drug often prescribed for pain management. Although opioids have powerful pain-relieving benefits, they are also highly addictive, can lead to adverse side effects like nausea and constipation, and can be lethal when overdosed.

With the current nationwide epidemic of opioid abuse, dependence, and fatalities, it's not enough to simply limit, taper, or discontinue the use of opioids to reduce reliance. People who are struggling with chronic pain need an effective alternative for pain management, and CBD and other cannabinoids can offer pain relief without the dangers posed by opioids.

Research has demonstrated that cannabinoids have far fewer side effects than opioids. They're not lethal. And, most importantly, cannabis is just as effective as opioids for relieving pain, if not more so. In fact, one study published in 2017 surveyed 2,897 medical cannabis patients. It found that 97 percent of the patients "strongly agreed/agreed" that they were able to decrease the amount of opioids they consumed when they also used cannabis. In addition, 81 percent "strongly agreed/agreed" that taking cannabis by itself was more effective at treating their condition than taking cannabis with opioids. The results were similar for those using cannabis with non-opioid-based pain medications. Overall, the "respondents overwhelmingly reported that cannabis provided relief on par with their other medications, but without the unwanted side effects."

Opioids vs. Cannabinoids	
High-dose opioids promote seizures.	Cannabinoids appear to have anti-convulsant activity.
Nausea and vomiting are common during opioid therapy.	Cannabinoids are used as an anti-emetic, especially for chemotherapy induced nausea and vomiting.
There is a chance of respiratory depression with opioid overdose.	There is no such risk with cannabinoids.

PART 2:
IS CBD OIL RIGHT FOR YOU?

CBD is an effective treatment for a wide range of medical conditions. In this section, we'll take a closer look at how CBD can be used to manage the symptoms of anxiety, chronic pain, migraines, and insomnia, and we'll delve into some of the most common questions I get from patients looking for relief from their symptoms. If you're suffering from anxiety, chronic pain, migraines, or insomnia, you may recognize your own experience in their stories.

WHAT CONDITIONS CAN BE TREATED WITH CBD?

CBD interacts with your body at a cellular level in a variety of ways, and has been shown to reduce inflammation, intercept pain signals to the brain, boost serotonin levels, dampen the flight-or-fight response, and help regulate sleep. Because of these qualities, there are many chronic medical conditions whose symptoms can be reduced or eliminated with the use of CBD. These include but are not limited to:

- Attention deficit disorder (ADD)
- Attention deficit hyperactivity disorder (ADHD)
- Back pain from bulging, herniated, or degenerative discs
- Back spasms
- Chemotherapy-induced neuropathy
- Diabetic neuropathy
- Epilepsy
- Generalized anxiety disorder
- Insomnia (mild to moderate)
- Menstrual cramps
- Migraines

- Multiple sclerosis
- Nerve pain from Lyme disease
- Obsessive-compulsive disorder (OCD)
- Panic disorder
- Parkinson's disease
- Post-traumatic stress disorder (PTSD)
- Sciatica
- Seizures
- Social anxiety
- Tension headaches
- Trigeminal neuralgia

On the next several pages, we'll look at some of the conditions that I most frequently treat, and what the research says about using CBD to treat them.

CBD for Anxiety

Dr. Patel,

I have paralyzing anxiety. It's mainly caused by stress at work. I manage a team of 17 and the deadlines are constantly looming.

At the end of the day, I go to bed hoping that I'll sleep soundly. But, more often than not, I lie awake for hours on end. My mind races nonstop with one worry after the next.

Some days it's so bad, I've had to call out of work. My heart races, I struggle to breathe, the room spins, and the sheets are soaked in sweat. Once, I ended up in the emergency room thinking I was having a heart attack. It turned out to be a panic attack.

My doctor prescribed Lexapro and Xanax. The Lexapro is killing my sex drive, and I'm having to use the Xanax more and more frequently in higher and higher doses. Addiction runs in my family and I'm not looking to head down that path.

I've read about CBD oil helping with anxiety, but I'm not sure about it, so I figured I'd ask a doctor.

Desperate,
Joe
Palo Alto, CA

I can really sympathize with patients like Joe. As a type-A in a very demanding profession, I know that anxiety can be totally and completely debilitating. But, there's hope, especially with the help of CBD.

WHAT THE RESEARCH SAYS...

Back in 2011, some researchers set to the task of looking at the effects of CBD on anxiety—specifically social anxiety. Half the participants were given CBD, and the other half were given placebo.

Participants were told they had two minutes to prepare a four-minute speech and that the speech would be recorded on video and then analyzed. Public speaking gives most people anxiety, so you can imagine how stressful this situation was for the participants already suffering from social anxiety.

However, you'll be pleasantly surprised to learn that the participants treated with CBD fared really well. Treatment with CBD significantly reduced anxiety, cognitive impairment, and discomfort. It led the researchers to conclude that a single dose of CBD could reduce the anxiety caused by public speaking in patients with social anxiety.

PATIENT RESULTS

My patients have reported that CBD works quite well to relieve anxiety. Patients feel more calm and more relaxed. They say CBD eases their anxiety in a way that allows them to function. They no longer feel paralyzed by the anxiety. The racing thoughts they have while lying in bed disappear, allowing them to fall asleep easily, stay asleep for a good seven to eight hours, and wake up well rested. Better rested, patients are able to take on the challenges of work with greater focus.

Most importantly, CBD helps to improve patients' relationships with their loved ones. Relieved of anxiety, they are no longer chronically tired, obsessively worried, or easily irritated. They show up as a better person for their family and friends.

Those who experience a very severe form of anxiety—panic attacks—report results ranging from complete elimination of their panic attacks to a reduction in the number and severity of the panic attacks.

In addition, patients report that they are able to eliminate or significantly reduce the dose and number of their prescription medications, such as SSRIs (selective serotonin reuptake inhibitors) and benzodiazepines. A select few find they have to continue to take their prescriptions medications; however, they experience greater relief of anxiety by combining the use of their prescription medications with CBD.

Patients also find that CBD is preferable to prescription medications due to its immediate effect and lack of unpleasant side effects.

CBD for Muscle Pain

Dr. Patel,

I need your help with my back pain. My back went out a while ago while lifting a heavy box. The pain came out of nowhere. It felt like a sharp knife stabbing through my back. It was so painful I couldn't move. I was on the couch for a couple days before I could get moving again, and the pain hasn't left me since. I still feel a "knot" in that same spot in my back, and that area cramps up when I sit or stand for a really long time or overexert myself.

Getting out of bed is a struggle. I wake up with a really stiff back. It's difficult to bend or stand. Meetings at work are a struggle. I have to continuously stand up to stretch my back. On long drives, I have to repeatedly make stops to stretch my back.

I've tried everything I can think of to relieve my back pain. I started by applying ice packs and heating pads. I went for some massages. I tried over-the-counter pain relievers, and I was prescribed a muscle relaxant, Baclofen, but it made me feel really drowsy, dizzy, and tired.

I need help. I've heard of people using CBD oil for back pain. What sort of results can I expect?

Regards,
Bob
Millburn, NJ

Back pain is one of the common conditions I've treated with CBD oil. Patients' symptoms can run the gamut from spasms to cramping or stiffness and even spasticity (a severe form of muscle cramps that affects the entire body). I've had patients who were once active go from limiting to completely quitting their favorite physical activities. It even impacts their personal and professional lives.

Many of the people who come to me for guidance on how to use CBD oil for their back pain have tried every other treatment they can think of. And more often than not, when nothing else helps, the CBD oil does.

WHAT THE RESEARCH SAYS...

While there hasn't been a tremendous amount of research on the effects of CBD on muscle pain, medical reports have shown CBD has been effective in reducing muscle pain.

In 2016, Dr. Amanda Morrow published a medical report on a case in which CBD was used to treat spasticity. The patient in this particular case suffered a spinal cord injury from a diving accident. His spasticity was so severe that he had a pump inserted in his abdomen to deliver on-demand medication, Baclofen, to relax his muscles.

At some point, the patient began to integrate CBD oil into his treatment. Over the course of three months, he was able to reduce his use of the muscle relaxant by 36 percent, and he reported excellent spasticity relief. He reported no adverse side effects from the CBD, including cognitive changes. He continued working full time and safely parenting his one-year-old child.

PATIENT RESULTS

In my practice, I've treated countless patients struggling with back pain. They've reported that CBD oil either dulls or completely eliminates their back pain. The reduction in pain depends on the level of pain they experienced before treatment. For patients with severe pain, the pain drops to a moderate level. For patients with moderate pain, the pain drops to a mild level. For those who start off with mild pain, CBD is often enough to completely eliminate their pain.

I also see a reduction in the frequency and duration of symptoms. Some patients have reported that they don't experience quite as many muscles spasms or as much cramping, stiffness, or spasticity. Others have reported that their spasms, cramping, stiffness, and spasticity doesn't last as long when using CBD oil.

Overall, with their pain better managed, patients are able to engage in activities like driving a car, sitting at a desk, or flying on a plane. They're also able to sleep through the night without awakening from the pain. Some patients even managed to completely come off the pharmaceutical drugs they were taking and use just the CBD oil on an as-needed basis to help manage their back pain.

CBD for Nerve Pain

Dr. Patel,

I've had diabetes for a while, and now I'm experiencing some really awful pain in my legs and feet from nerve damage caused by the diabetes. At first, I was having pain here and there and didn't make much of it, but now, it's turned into a nuisance that won't leave me alone, night or day. It's relentless.

At the start of the day, much of what I feel is numbness, but as the day goes on, the numbness turns into a feeling of pins and needles prickling my legs and feet. Sometimes I feel like my legs and feet are on fire. I wake up in the middle of the night with a feeling of electric shocks shooting down my legs. It's painful even to have socks on.

After a lot of trial and error with medication, I've been using gabapentin to take the edge off. Every once in a while, it allows me to have a good day, but I have to say that most days are still bad days.

I'm still searching for a solution which can help me turn most of my bad days into good days. I've been putting my life on hold because this pain. Have you found that CBD oil helps patients with neuropathy?

Warm regards,
Samantha,
Los Angeles, CA

I get questions about nerve pain, or *neuropathy,* from a lot of patients. Some, like Samantha, suffer from neuropathy that stems from diabetes, but there are many other causes of neuropathy, including:

- Nerve compression (sciatica, for example)
- Multiple sclerosis
- Chemotherapy
- Surgical damage
- Carpal tunnel syndrome
- Lyme disease
- Complex regional pain syndrome (CRPS)
- Poor circulation

I've also treated cases of idiopathic neuropathy, which is when the cause of the neuropathy is unknown.

WHAT THE RESEARCH SAYS...

One group of researchers pooled together data from five different studies on the impact of CBD on neuropathic pain in 41 patients. They found that a placebo reduced pain by 0.8 points on average, while CBD decreased pain by 1.5 points on average. It's important to note that in most of these studies, patients in the placebo group were allowed to receive rescue drugs for pain and were allowed to increase the doses of those pain drugs. In addition, the pain relief from CBD was sustained during the 6- to 10-week follow-up period.

PATIENT RESULTS

Chronic pain is one the most common conditions that I treat, and neuropathy is one of the most common causes of chronic pain.

CBD oil helps to either dull or eliminate patients' pain, depending on the patient's starting level of pain. Those with severe pain may have their pain reduced to a mild or moderate level. Those starting with mild or moderate pain may find their pain completely eliminated.

For some patients, CBD helps to reduce the use of their prescription pain medications. They're able to reduce the dosages of the medications, or they find they can cut back on the number of medications they're taking. In some cases, patients are able to completely eliminate prescription pain medications and manage their pain with the use of CBD oil alone. Overall, the vast majority of my patients report that the CBD oil works as well as, if not better than, opioids, but without the side effects.

Opioids are a group of drugs that interact with opioid receptors. They are commonly prescribed for pain relief, but cause unwanted adverse side effects and are potentially lethal.

CBD for Migraines

Dr. Patel,

I need more info on using CBD oil for migraine headaches. I've suffered from migraines for over 20 years, and they're getting worse.

I usually get one migraine a week and it can last up to three days. The headaches can go from a throbbing to a pounding pain pretty quickly, and are without fail accompanied by nausea and vomiting.

I'm left completely debilitated on these days. All the important things that I have to get done are left to the wayside. I'm locked in my room with the shades drawn.

Prescription medications tend to give me really uncomfortable side effects, or they just don't work. Right now, I use Imitrex to stop the migraines, but if I don't catch the headache at just the right moment, then I've completely lost the opportunity to stop the migraine, and I just have to live with it for the next two to three days.

Otherwise, over-the-counter pain medications don't come anywhere close to touching the pain.

So, what do you think? CBD oil? Yay or nay?

Regards,
Hannah
Atherton, CA

I've heard from thousands of patients like Hannah over the years, and I know that living with chronic migraines is a miserable experience. You're certainly not alone in your struggle with migraines. Migraines affect 12 percent of the general population—that's close to 1 in every 10 people you meet.

WHAT THE RESEARCH SAYS...

There's not much in the way of research on the effects of CBD on migraines, so let's just go ahead dive straight into the results my patients have experienced with the use of CBD.

PATIENT RESULTS

CBD has helped patients by reducing the severity, duration, and frequency of migraine headaches. When patients rated their migraine pain on a scale of 1–10, with 10 being most severe, on average those with a pain level of 7–9 reported that CBD helped to bring their pain down to a 1–3. When starting with a pain level of 4–6, more often than not the CBD eliminated the pain.

Patients have also reported that CBD reduced how long their migraines lasted. When using triptans, such as Imitrex, they absolutely had to catch the migraine at just the right moment; otherwise they'd have to bear the pain for two or three days. With CBD, patients reported that they weren't limited to using it within a certain window of time. And when they did use the CBD, the migraines typically resolved within about an hour.

Patients have reported that prior to using CBD, they were having migraines on average about one to three times per month. With the use of CBD, they began to have migraines much less frequently. On average, they reported having migraines about once every three to six months, if that. In best-case scenarios, patients reported not experiencing any migraines at all when they used CBD in a preventative way.

Triptans are a class of medication commonly used to treat migraines. They work by stimulating serotonin receptors.

CBD for Sleep

Dr. Patel,

I can't sleep. I have a hard time falling asleep. I can't stay asleep. And I wake up feeling like a total wreck. I've suffered from insomnia for over 25 years, and I think I've tried everything under the sun to find relief.

Over-the-counter sleep aids, like Unisom and ZzzQuil, have left me feeling hungover the next morning. Melatonin doesn't work anymore. I took Ambien for several years, but that stuff has some pretty scary side effects. Even when Ambien did help me sleep, I never woke up feeling well rested. I'd walk around feeling like a zombie the following day.

Recently, I was telling a friend about my trouble sleeping. He happened to have some CBD oil on hand. I tried some, and I have to say I was definitely surprised. I had the best sleep I've had in years.

Was it just a fluke? Does CBD oil really help with sleep?

Sincerely,
Bill
New York, NY

I'm all too familiar with the struggle to sleep. As an overworked medical resident, I found myself wired. There were weeks when I'd work 90 hours in five days and would be on my feet for 30 hours at a time, but I couldn't get in a wink of sleep when I got home. I even got a script for Ambien from my doctor, but after reading up on the side effects, I never ended up filling the script. Looking back, I wish I had access to CBD. It would've definitely helped.

WHAT THE RESEARCH SAYS...

A study published in 1981 looked at the effects of CBD on people suffering from insomnia in Sao Paulo, Brazil from 1972 to 1981. For this study, participants were selected based on their history of difficult sleeping. They had trouble falling asleep (at least one hour) and experienced poor sleep throughout the night. Over five weeks, the participants were given a capsule that contained either CBD, glucose, or nitrazepam (a minor tranquilizer) at night. In the morning, they had to complete a questionnaire. The participants who were given CBD reported sleeping more than seven hours, having fewer interruptions of sleep, and getting a good night's sleep overall.

PATIENT RESULTS

In my practice, I've found that I need to treat patients with mild or moderate insomnia much differently from patients with severe insomnia. Those with mild or moderate insomnia fare better with CBD oil, whereas those with severe insomnia don't. I've also found that patients who have difficulty falling asleep need a different treatment approach from patients who have difficulty staying asleep.

In terms of results, I've had patients report that they fall asleep more easily, stay asleep throughout the night, and fall back asleep easily if they wake up in the middle of the night. On average, they get about seven to eight hours of sleep per night, and wake up well rested rather than groggy.

When it comes to prescription medications, generally those with mild or moderate insomnia are able to eliminate the use of over-the-counter sleeping aids. Some patients on prescription sleeping aids are able to eliminate their use completely, while other patients find that they don't rely on them as much, and only use them when they don't have access to CBD oil.

USE WITH CAUTION

While CBD can be an effective treatment for many, there are some people who should proceed with caution.

Pregnant or breastfeeding women: There is a lack of conclusive data on the effects of CBD on a developing fetus or a growing breastfed baby. However, some evidence suggests that CBD may cause developmental toxicity in animals, including increased fetal mortality in rats and decreased fetal body weights in rabbits.

In addition, CBD can increase levels of anadamide, a cannabinoid that occurs naturally in the body. One study found that high levels of anadamide were associated with failure to achieve an ongoing pregnancy after in vitro fertilization.

In general, it's best to avoid unnecessary exposure to anything that's potentially harmful during pregnancy. Having said that, you can consult with your physician, who will take into consideration the medical benefits of CBD along with your needs, as well as any potential adverse effects on a developing fetus or breastfed baby.

Children: Clinical trials of Epidiolex established CBD as safe and effective in children two years of age and older. However, due to the differences in dosing needs for children, it is best administered under the care of a physician.

Patients with liver disease: Elevated liver enzymes levels have been reported with the CBD-based drug Epidiolex, most commonly when used in conjunction with valproate, a seizure medication. Though the liver injury was generally mild, it raises the possibility of rare, but more severe liver injury.

A BETTER ALTERNATIVE

You now know that there are many, many different medical conditions for which CBD is effective. It's evident from both the research and the clinical results I've witnessed as a physician. We're not just talking about a medical case here and there—it's patient after patient after patient with the same medical conditions, reporting the same results with the use of CBD.

The vast majority of my patients with headaches and migraines, muscle pain, nerve pain, anxiety, and sleeplessness have benefited from the use of CBD. Many of these patients have come to me seeking CBD oil as a last resort after having tried a variety of conventional medications. For many people, CBD oil proved to be a more effective and safer alternative to prescription and over-the-counter medications. I'd even go so far to say that CBD oil is a much more suitable alternative to the over-the-counter medications that are commonly used to treat pain and sleeplessness, such as acetaminophen (Tylenol), ibuprofen (Advil), and diphenhydramine (Unisom). So, is CBD right for you? It could very well be the answer you're looking for.

PART 3:
HOW TO BUY CBD OIL

....

Now that you know how helpful CBD can be in treating various conditions, you probably want to know where you can get some. The answer is somewhat contingent on where you live. Depending on your state of residence, you may be able to purchase CBD oil at a state-licensed dispensary, through an online retailer, or from a brick-and-mortar store, such as a food co-op or natural foods store. States where marijuana is legal for recreational or medical use will have more options for purchasing CBD, but at the time of this writing, most US residents have options for buying some form of CBD. The one place you won't find CBD products—at least, not yet—is your local pharmacy.

So, you've found a CBD product to purchase. Before you hand over your money, take the time to do your research and make sure you're buying a reputable product. This section covers the types of available CBD products, what to look for on the product label, and the importance of obtaining lab results.

OPTIONS VARY BY STATE

Remember that CBD can come from two sources: it can come from marijuana, and it can come from hemp. Laws surrounding CBD vary on a state-by-state basis depending on its source. In the United States, they fall into four categories:

- Both marijuana- and hemp-derived CBD are legal.
- Marijuana-derived CBD is legal, but hemp-derived CBD is not.
- Hemp-derived CBD is legal, but marijuana-derived CBD is not.
- Neither marijuana- nor hemp-derived CBD are legal.

If you live in a state with state-licensed dispensaries, there's more oversight and regulation of the products sold. Every state has their own quality control standards. I recommend checking out your state department of public health website for further information on the rules and regulations surrounding CBD.

TYPES OF CBD PRODUCTS

Although CBD oil is one of the most common and well-known formulations of CBD, there are CBD products available in other forms as well. Let's look at some of the ways CBD is sold and used.

Oils (Tinctures): Oils, also called *tinctures,* are likely the most familiar form of CBD. They are made by combining CBD extract with a carrier oil. An oil (or tincture) comes in a bottle with a dropper or a spray-top cap. Some oils may be flavored to make them more palatable.

On the package, an oil may be identified as "CBD oil," "hemp oil," or "hemp extract oil." However, do not mistake a product made with hemp seeds for a CBD product. Hemp seeds on their own contain insignificant levels of CBD, and hemp seed oil, which can be purchased for culinary applications, does not contain significant levels of CBD.

Topicals: Often found in the form of salves, balms, or ointments, topicals are applied to the affected area. Topicals have a myriad of benefits when it comes to skin conditions and muscle and joint pain. A variety of bases are used to create the topicals, the most common of which are shea butter and coconut oil.

Capsules: CBD extract is combined with a carrier oil and housed in a capsule. With a capsule, the dose of CBD is fixed, so it's a limiting form when trying to tweak and determine your appropriate dose.

Vapes: The CBD extract is housed in a cartridge that attaches to a vape pen, giving you the option to inhale CBD, similar to an e-cigarette.

Edibles: The CBD extract (combined with a carrier oil) is used to create an edible food product, such as chocolates or gummies.

Concentrates: These are CBD extracts that are not combined with a carrier oil or a base. As the name implies, they are a more concentrated substance with a thick, paste-like consistency.

READING THE LABEL

When considering a CBD product for purchase, read the label or product description carefully, and be sure you understand the information presented.

Amount of CBD

Labels should tell you the amount of CBD in the product. There are two spots on the package to look for the total amount of CBD. The first is the "Supplement Facts" panel. Here you'll find the amount of CBD provided as milligrams per serving.

Otherwise, the concentration of CBD may be listed anywhere else on the package. In this case, the total amount of CBD in the product is just provided outright. When provided outright, you'll find the total milligrams of CBD in the product, not the amount of CBD per serving. (Note that the amount of THC may not be listed, as it's not the active ingredient in the product.)

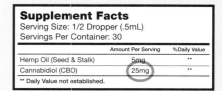

Supplement Facts
Serving Size: 1/2 Dropper (.5mL)
Servings Per Container: 30

	Amount Per Serving	%Daily Value
Hemp Oil (Seed & Stalk)	5mg	**
Cannabidiol (CBD)	25mg	**
** Daily Value not established.		

This product has 25mg of CBD per .5mL serving, and there are 30 servings per container, so the total amount of CBD is 750mg in the 15mL container.

To compare the concentration of CBD in different CBD goods, look at products of equivalent volumes. The concentration in the most common form of CBD — the oil — can range from 250 milligrams per fluid ounce to about 1,000 milligrams per fluid ounce.

Now, here's a really important point to take note of: some labels simply don't state the amount of CBD anywhere on the label, which doesn't really serve you, the consumer. You need to know exactly what you're putting in your body and how much of it. Taking too little CBD gives you no medical benefit, and taking too much CBD can result in adverse side effects, even if they're not serious.

A well-labeled CBD oil should include the exact amount of CBD, whether it's the total amount of CBD outright or the amount of CBD per serving.

Avoid Products with Unclear Labeling

Supplement Facts
Serving Size: 0.6ml (1 Dropper Full)
Servings Per Container: 25

	Amount Per % Daily Serving
Calories	9
Calories from Fat	9
Total Fat	1g
Phytocannabinoid Hemp Oil	30mg**

*Percent Daily Values are based on 2,000 calorie diet
** Daily Value not established.

Ingredients: Hemp seed oil and PCR Hemp oil

Supplement Facts
Serving Size: 1 Dropper Full (1ml)
Servings Per Container: 25

Amount Per Serving	% Daily Value**
Calories 9	
Calories from Fat 9	
Total Fat 1g	2%
Saturated Fat 0g	
Hemp Extract 33mg	**

*Percent Daily Values are based on 2,000 calorie diet
** Daily Value not established.

Supplement Facts
Serving Size: 1 Dropper Full (1ml)
Servings Per Container: 25

Amount Per Serving %DV**	
Calories 9 Calories from Fat 9	

	% Daily Value**
Total Fat	0.9g
Linoleic Acid	405mg
Alpha Linoleic Acid	135mg
Oleic Acid	90mg

*Percent Daily Values are based on 2,000 calorie diet
** Daily Value not established.

This label indicates the amount of "Phytocannabinoid Hemp Oil" per serving. The word *phytocannabinoid* encompasses over 100 different cannabinoids made by hemp. This might include CBD, but you don't know for sure.

This label indicates the amount of "Hemp Extract" per serving. The word *extract* encompasses all the chemicals made by hemp in its concentrated form. You don't know if there is CBD in the product, or how much.

This particular label gives you no information whatsoever. There may be CBD in this product. There may not be. The world may never know. Don't bother considering a product that's labeled like this.

Serving Size

Now, I want to turn your attention to the serving size, which is also part of the supplement facts panel. It's important to understand that the amount listed as one serving is just an estimate. It may or may not be the right serving size for you. For some, that amount might be too much. For others, that amount might be too little. In my experience treating patients, I've found that the serving size, or dose, varies greatly from person to person. You can use the serving size listed on the label as a guide, but ultimately, it's best to work with an experienced doctor to figure out the dose that's right for you, especially if you're using CBD to treat a specific medical problem.

Isolate vs. Full Spectrum

Some CBD products are marketed using the terms "CBD isolate" or "full-spectrum CBD." I'll give you a very clear idea of what they mean so that you can be a smart consumer.

The term *full-spectrum* means that the product contains CBD plus all the other cannabinoids found in the hemp plant. Of course, this includes the trace amounts of THC, up to 0.3 percent. The terms "full-spectrum" and "whole plant" are often used interchangeably.

An *isolate,* as the name implies, contains just CBD that's been extracted from the hemp plant and is isolated from the other cannabinoids. The CBD is isolated using a process called *chromatography.* It's a separation method used to isolate a single chemical from a mixture. CBD products made with isolate CBD are typically labeled as "pure CBD."

Now, here's the all-important question: Which is more effective, full-spectrum CBD or isolate CBD? Research done on mice at Israel's Hebrew University showed that CBD in its full-spectrum form was far more effective than CBD as an isolate. One group of mice was administered CBD in its full-spectrum form, while another group of mice was given CBD as an isolate. The study found that far smaller doses of full-spectrum CBD were needed than isolate CBD to achieve the same pain-relieving effect. In other words, the mice got more bang for their buck with the full-spectrum CBD compared to the isolate CBD.

So, it's quite possible that CBD combined with the other phytocannabinoids, in full-spectrum form, may be more effective than on its own as an isolate.

Extract Solvents

In Part 1, we looked at the various ways CBD can be extracted from the hemp plant. Some of these extraction solvents are more desirable than others. Avoid CBD extracted using a hydrocarbon, which has been associated with increased health risks, even in small amounts. CBD extracted using carbon dioxide and ethanol are better options. CBD extracted in an oil may be acceptable as well, depending on your needs.

A Word of Caution

Because CBD is not subject to federal regulation, there's a chance that what you see on the label is not what you get. In 2015 and 2016, the FDA set out to test the CBD content of CBD oils from a variety of manufacturers. They found that in many cases, the product labels wildly misrepresented the actual CBD content of the product. Many of the tested CBD oils contained much less CBD than indicated on the label. In addition, some of the CBD oils contained more than 0.3 percent THC.

A 2017 study showed similar results. In this study, researchers tested 84 different CBD products from 31 different companies. According to their results:

- 42.85% of the products were underlabeled, meaning the CBD content in the product exceeded the labeled amount by more than 10 percent.

- 26.19% of the products were overlabeled, meaning the CBD content in the product was less than the labeled amount by more than 10 percent.

- Only 30.95% of the products were accurately labeled, meaning the CBD content of the product tested within 10 percent of labeled amount.

Interestingly, some types of products were more likely to be mislabeled than others. Vaporization liquid was the most frequently mislabeled, while oil was the product most frequently labeled accurately.

The risks of using a mislabeled product are relatively low, but may cause adverse effects. An overlabeled product (having less CBD than reported) won't work to alleviate symptoms, leading to a waste of your time and money. An underlabeled product (having more CBD than reported on the label) is not a great concern because CBD doesn't appear to have abuse liability or serious adverse consequences at high doses; however, it may cause side effects such as drowsiness. And, of course, a product with levels of THC higher 0.3 percent may cause an unwanted high.

How do you avoid purchasing a mislabeled product? The answer is to demand state-licensed, third-party lab tests that provide unbiased information about the content of the product.

LOOKING AT LAB RESULTS

Checking out the state-licensed, third-party lab test results is the single most important piece of due diligence you should do before you even consider buying any CBD product. Do not purchase a CBD product until you've seen the lab test results with your very own eyes. Ask the company selling the CBD product for the lab test results. If they can't provide lab test results, don't buy the product.

Before you dive into the nitty gritty of the lab test results, you'll want to look up the lab at which the CBD product was tested. It's better to have results from a lab that's licensed by the state. In order to obtain and maintain a license, labs are inspected and audited for proper testing practices and standards of performance. Further information can be found on the department of health website for the state in which the lab is located.

Amounts of CBD and THC

Lab test results will provide the actual amounts of CBD and THC in the CBD product. The amounts of CBD and THC are provided as percentages and/or as milligrams per gram. With the help of some mathematical calculations, you'll be able to compare the labeled CBD amount to the amount on the lab test results. Make sure the CBD oil has been tested for THC as well, to confirm that the level of THC does not exceed 0.3 percent. (The amount of THC may not be listed on the product label, as it's not one of the active ingredients in CBD products.)

Potency Report

Cannabinoid	%Weight	mg/g
CBD	2.5%	50.0
THC	.003%	1.0

When comparing the CBD product label to the lab results, be aware that 1g is approximately equal to 1mL.

Fungi and Bacteria

Bacteria and fungi that cause harm to humans aren't all that common on cannabis plants, and the CBD extraction process generally kills off and inactivates most fungi and bacteria and the toxins that they make. However, it is possible that a hemp or marijuana plant could be contaminated and that the bad bugs could make their way into CBD product.

For people with healthy immune systems, the most worrisome of these are *Salmonella* and *E. coli*, but people with compromised immune systems should also be concerned about *Pseudomonas aeruginosa* and *Aspergillus*. (At-risk people include those who are undergoing chemotherapy, those who have HIV/ AIDS, and those who are on immunosuppressants.) The best way to protect yourself against contaminated CBD product is to ask for the lab test results.

WHAT SHOULD THE LAB TESTS SAY?

Make sure that the CBD product has been tested for *Salmonella* and *E. coli,* and additionally for *Pseudomonas aeruginosa* and *Aspergillus* for those who have a compromised immune system. The amounts of fungi and bacteria should not exceed established limits, which are generally stated on the lab test results as colony forming unit (CFU) per gram (CFU/g). The CBD product should pass the lab test for every type of microbe that's screened.

Microbial Analysis Results

Test	CFU/gram Count	Limit(CFU/gram)	Pass/Fail
E. coli	ND	< 1	Pass
Salmonella	ND	< 1	Pass
Total Yeast & Mold	ND	< 10000	Pass

ND = not detected

Lab results should show that no fungi or bacteria were detected.

Pesticides

Like any crop, marijuana and hemp plants are susceptible to pests, and some farmers use pesticides to control unwanted pests on plants. Continual exposure to low doses of pesticides can cause them to accumulate in your body, usually in your fatty tissues. Over time, this accumulation can increase the likelihood of certain medical problems, including cancer, neuropathy, asthma, allergies, and degenerative diseases, such as Parkinson's, Alzheimer's, and multiple sclerosis.

Pesticides are especially a concern with concentrates, which is what CBD products essentially are. Based on extensive research, the Cannabis Safety Institute found that the mean levels of pesticide residues found in cannabis concentrates is higher than that found in cannabis flowers. If you think about it, this makes sense. The processes that concentrate the cannabinoids also concentrate the pesticides. Because CBD products are made from a series of processes that concentrate the CBD, it's also likely that any pesticides used to grow the hemp are also likely to be concentrated.

REGULATIONS ON PESTICIDE TESTING

Rules and regulations related to the cannabis family of plants vary from state to state. While some states specify which pesticides to test for and how to test for them, other states remain silent about pesticide use on cannabis. According the Cannabis Safety Institute, even when rules and regulations for pesticide testing are in place, they may be based on inappropriate screening techniques or invalid protocols and may be arbitrary at best. Given that testing for pesticides on cannabis is in its infancy, states are continually having to visit and revisit their rules and regulations on pesticide testing.

At the end of the day, it's possible you may be sold a CBD oil labeled "chemical-free," "pesticide-free," "organic," or "all-natural," when, in fact, that's just not the case. The best way to ensure that your product is free of pesticides is to look at the lab results.

WHAT SHOULD THE LAB TESTS SAY?

The Cannabis Safety Institute recommends testing for 123 target pesticides, which can be found on their website. When you look at the lab test results, check that the product has been tested for as many of the target pesticides listed by the Cannabis Safety Institute as possible, especially bifenazate and myclobutanil. The amounts of the pesticides should not exceed established limits, which are generally stated on the lab test results as either parts per million or parts per billion.

Pesticide Screening Results

Pesticide	Result (ppm)	Pass/Fail
Bifenazate	ND	Pass
Myclobutanil	ND	Pass
Azoxystrobin	ND	Pass

ND = not detected

The CBD product should pass the lab test for every pesticide that's screened.

Heavy Metals

As plants grow, they accumulate metals. These metals may occur naturally in the soil and water, or they may be artificially introduced through the use of fertilizers and pesticides or even industrialization and power generation. Plants in the cannabis family are known as *hyperaccumulators* because they have a strong affinity for accumulating heavy metals. This can be problematic, because heavy metals in high concentration are hazardous to human health. They're not broken down easily and can accumulate in the body instead. They can cause a variety of health problems, including cancer, brain damage, and nerve damage.

WHAT SHOULD THE LAB TESTS SAY?

Your CBD product should be tested for arsenic, lead, cadmium, and mercury. The limits of detection vary based on the method used to detect the heavy metals. The limits of detection should be provided on the lab test results, and the CBD product should pass the lab test for each type of heavy metal.

Heavy Metal Screening Results

Heavy Metal	Result (ppm)	Pass/Fail
Arsenic	ND	Pass
Lead	ND	Pass
Cadmium	ND	Pass
Mercury	ND	Pass

ND = not detected

Lab results should show that no heavy metals were detected.

Residual Solvents

In some cases, the extraction method used to make the CBD product might leave behind residual solvents. This is particularly a concern for CBD products made with hydrocarbons, because these pose potential health risks. If the CBD product you're purchasing was made with hydrocarbon, get the lab test results. The amount of residual solvent should not exceed the established limits, which are generally stated on the lab test results. The CBD product should pass the lab test for every residual solvent that's screened.

Residual Solvent Analysis Results

Solvent	Result (ppm)	Limit	Pass/Fail
n-Butane	ND	< 5000	Pass
Hexane	ND	< 290	Pass
Heptane	ND	< 5000	Pass

ND = not detected

A screen for residual solvents should show that none were detected.

Lab Results Mitigate Risk

Overall, there are risks that come with using CBD products, just like any other prescription or over-the-counter medication, but with due diligence, those risks can be mitigated. The key is to ask the right questions and know how to get the answers you're looking for. Seek out manufacturers that provide state-licensed, third-party lab testing, and make sure the product you're purchasing is labeled accurately.

PART 4:
HOW TO USE CBD

More often than not, people expect to buy a CBD product, take some, and immediately feel relief, just like that. Unfortunately, that's not quite how it works. As with any medication, there's a very specific way to take CBD for every medical condition.

Over the years, I've developed a five-step process—The Patel Protocol—to help patients determine how to best use CBD. In this section, you'll find a broad overview of the steps. For a more in-depth look at using CBD to treat specific medical conditions, visit DrRachnaPatel.com. There you'll find protocols by medical condition that will guide you through the nuances of each one.

STEP 1: **DETERMINE THE RIGHT COMBINATION OF CANNABINOIDS**

The first step is to figure out which combination of cannabinoids to use to get the best results. Some medical conditions do better with more THC. Some medical conditions need both THC and CBD. And then there are conditions that benefit from more CBD (see Part 2).

The CBD can come from marijuana or it can come from hemp, so you can use either cannabis oil or hemp oil. Both fall under the general category of CBD oils.

Hemp oil, by default, has more CBD than THC; more specifically, it has less than 0.3 percent THC, making it a desirable option for conditions that are benefited by higher levels of CBD.

With cannabis oil, the lab test results have to be closely examined to figure out just how much more CBD there is relative to THC. For conditions benefited by CBD, obviously, the greater the amount of CBD relative to THC, the better.

Benefited by High CBD	Need Some Amount of THC
• Migraines and headaches	• Nausea and vomiting
• Muscle pain, such as back spasms	• Lack of appetite
• Nerve pain, such as back pain caused by sciatica, neuropathy caused by diabetes or chemotherapy, and even trigeminal neuralgia	• Autoimmune conditions, such as psoriasis, rheumatoid arthritis, Crohn's disease, ulcerative colitis, and lupus
• Anxiety, including obsessive-compulsive disorder (OCD), post-traumatic stress disorder (PTSD), attention deficit disorder (ADD), attention deficit hyperactivity disorder (ADHD), and panic disorder	• Severe nerve pain, such as pain caused by shingles and spinal stenosis
• Mild or moderate insomnia	• Severe insomnia, when sleep without medication is impossible

STEP 2: **SELECT THE BEST DELIVERY METHOD**

The next step is to select the delivery method or methods that will work most effectively for your medical condition.

Sublingual: With the sublingual option, drops of CBD oil are placed under the tongue, where they can easily be absorbed by the blood vessels located there. I recommend a flavored CBD oil to make the taste more tolerable. CBD oils used under the tongue are medically referred to as *sublingual CBD oil,* but colloquially are called *tinctures.*

Ingestion: There's also the option of eating CBD. You can buy prepared products, such as chocolates or gummies made with CBD oil, or you can make your own. See Part 5 for a selection of sweet and savory CBD recipes.

Topical: The form of CBD oil that's used on the skin. Topicals can be used to alleviate symptoms caused by medical conditions of the skin or to alleviate certain types of pain. In my practice, CBD topicals have been particularly effective in helping to relieve localized muscle pain.

There are a couple ways to go about this option. Topicals made with CBD can be purchased, or CBD oil can be directly applied to the affected area. You can also make your own CBD topicals using the spa and wellness recipes in Part 5.

Inhalation: There are two ways to inhale—smoke or vaporize. Smoking entails heating something to the point that it burns, while vaping involves heating something below its burning point.

It's not a common practice to smoke CBD, and I don't recommend it anyway. It creates harmful toxins and is pretty much like breathing in pollution. However, it is a common practice to vaporize CBD oil. Research shows that by avoiding the process of burning, vaping significantly reduces the amounts of harmful toxins that are produced. Typically, CBD oil is vaped in a device known as a vape pen. It comes with a cartridge filled with CBD oil.

Rectal: This may be an unexpected option, but it is an effective delivery method for people who are unable to inhale or consume CBD. It comes in the form of a suppository.

Important Considerations

Keep in mind that some delivery methods can work very effectively for certain medical conditions and not so well for others. For example, the external use of CBD in the form of a topical doesn't work to relieve anxiety, and the internal use of CBD in the form of edibles may not be the best choice for a localized area of muscle pain.

Another important consideration is your medical history. Over the years, I've treated a number of patients who have undergone gastric bypass surgery, a procedure in which the size of the stomach is reduced to induce weight loss. These patients did not absorb edibles well, so we had to use alternative delivery methods. As another example, for a patient with a lung condition, like asthma, vaporization is not an appropriate delivery method, as it could worsen the patient's symptoms.

Also consider the nature of the symptoms. Vaporization, for example, is particularly helpful in situations that require immediate relief, such as with episodes of breakthrough pain. When inhaled, you'll notice the effects of CBD within 5 to 10 minutes.

STEP 3: **FIGURE OUT THE RIGHT DOSE**

"Take one dropper of CBD per day," or "Take X milligrams of CBD per day," are some of the most common CBD dosage recommendations you'll find on labels. While these can definitely be doses, you don't know if it's the right dose for you. These CBD dose recommendations don't take into account the concentration of CBD, your body's biochemistry, the condition being treated, or the severity of your symptoms.

It's important to understand that CBD has a subtherapeutic, therapeutic, and supratherapeutic range of dosing. A subtherapeutic dose is too low and will not help to relieve your symptoms. A supratherapeutic dose is too high and can cause side effects. The aim is for a therapeutic dose. It's the dose that's just right. It's the dose where the CBD is helping to relieve symptoms without any adverse side effects.

Everyone is different, and everyone reacts differently to specific CBD dosages—there isn't a "one size fits all" dosage. What works for one person may not be enough for another person or too much for someone else. In my years treating patients, I've found that the therapeutic dose of CBD oil varies greatly from person to person. I've had patients use anywhere from a fraction of a milligram of CBD to a couple hundred milligrams of CBD.

As the dosage of CBD differs for each person, it's best to start with a small dose and gradually increase the dose until the desired result is achieved. Take notes to document how much CBD you took. Remember, the less CBD that's taken to get relief, the better. There's no point in taking more CBD than needed. For additional guidance, consult a physician who has experience dosing CBD or visit DrRachnaPatel.com.

STEP 4: **DETERMINE FREQUENCY OF USE**

Multiple factors play a role in determining how often to take the CBD, including how well the CBD is absorbed, where it's distributed in your body, how quickly it's metabolized, and the rate at which CBD is eliminated. Because each individual has unique biochemistry, some people need more frequent dosing, while others need less frequent dosing. For example, in patients with liver disease, metabolism of drugs in general slows down, including metabolism of CBD. This means patients with liver disease who take CBD need to have the frequency of dosing adjusted accordingly.

The nature of your medical condition also matters. Some people experience symptoms episodically and need longer intervals between doses. Others experience symptoms on an ongoing basis and need to use CBD more regularly with much shorter intervals between doses. For example, in patients with migraines, the interval of dosing varies by the frequency and duration of migraines they experience over a set period of time.

Be methodical about determining your frequency of use. Take notes to document when you took the CBD.

STEP 5: **TRACK YOUR USE**

There's a science to figuring out how much medication to take and how often to take it. One of the most important tools utilized as a part of this process is tracking. Tracking provides a method to the madness. Tracking your patterns of CBD consumption provides you with a means of observing the effects of CBD on your symptoms. In turn, this information can be used to further refine the use of CBD to attain the desired result.

Strength of CBD Product:

Symptoms Prior to Using CBD Product:

Date and Time	Amount Taken	Effect on Symptoms

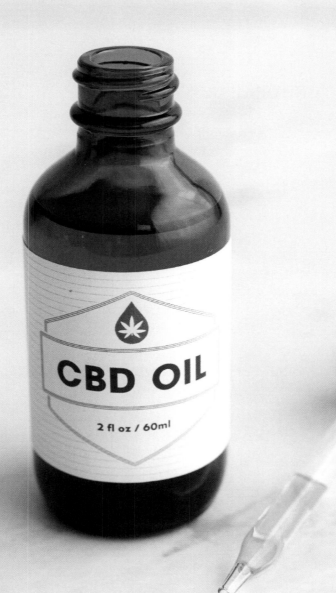

THE FAQS ABOUT CBD

Still have questions? Here you'll find answers to some of the most commonly asked questions about CBD that aren't covered elsewhere in the book.

CAN I TAKE CBD WITH OTHER MEDICATIONS?

Overall, CBD is relatively safe, well tolerated, and carries fewer risks of adverse drug interactions than many other commonly prescribed drugs.

However, it's important to know that CBD can make some prescription medications more effective, thereby helping to reduce the need for that drug. CBD can also make some drugs less effective, thereby necessitating changes in how the drug is administered.

If you're taking prescription medications, the best way to learn about specific drug interactions is by working with a knowledgeable and experienced physician. He or she can take a look at the specific medications you're taking and tell you what you should and shouldn't be worried about when it comes to taking CBD with your medications.

DOES CBD OIL HAVE SIDE EFFECTS?

Side effects are a big concern for many people. The great news is that CBD has not been shown to cause many of the negative side effects common to prescription medications. In 2017, a group of researchers sifted through medical study upon medical study and determined that CBD has not been found to cause changes in heart rate, breathing, blood pressure, or body temperature. It has no effect on psychomotor function (skills related to movement and coordination), and it doesn't affect learning (like the ability to recall words). It doesn't cause changes in appetite or weight, and it doesn't cause depression or psychosis. CBD also doesn't cause any of the negative side effects commonly associated with marijuana.

So, what side effects does CBD cause? The most commonly reported side effects are fatigue, tiredness, and sleepiness. The severity of these is dose-dependent. When used correctly, it's unlikely that you'll experience any adverse effects from CBD. In the case that you do, adjusting how much, when, or how often you use the CBD oil will likely help.

WILL I FAIL A DRUG TEST IF I TAKE A CBD PRODUCT?

It depends on the composition of cannabinoids in the product you've used. If the product does not contain any THC, then you would not test positive for marijuana or marijuana metabolite.

However, if the product does contain THC—no matter the amount—then you could test positive for marijuana or marijuana metabolite. The only CBD product in which no THC should be detected is a CBD isolate. Any other CBD product will have some amount of THC in it.

IS CBD ADDICTIVE?

Nope! It comes straight from the horse's mouth: according to the National Institute on Drug Abuse, "CBD appears to be a safe drug with no addictive effects."

CAN I BRING A CBD PRODUCT ON A PLANE?

It's probably not a good idea. According to the Transportation Security Administration (TSA), "Possession of marijuana and cannabis-infused products, such as cannabidiol (CBD) oil, is illegal under federal law. TSA officers are required to report any suspected violations of law, including possession of marijuana- and cannabis-infused products. TSA's screening procedures are focused on security and are designed to detect potential threats to aviation and passengers. Accordingly, TSA security officers do not search for marijuana or other illegal drugs, but in the event a substance that appears to be marijuana or a cannabis-infused product is observed during security screening, TSA will refer the matter to a law enforcement officer."

In other words, TSA agents aren't specifically looking for CBD, but they will report it to authorities if they find it. So, fly with CBD at your own risk.

CAN MY PET USE CBD PRODUCTS?

There are a certainly veterinarians out there who treat pets with CBD products. Your veterinarian can advise you on which CBD product to use and how much and how often to administer it based on your pet's condition.

PART 5:
CBD RECIPES

In this section, you'll find recipes for beverages, sweet and savory dishes, and a variety of spa and wellness products, all of which can be made with a commercially prepared, unflavored CBD oil.

Before making a recipe, determine the right dose of CBD for you, and use that as a serving. Too much oil may affect the flavor or consistency of the finished dish or product, so take care not to use more than the amount called for in the recipe. If the dose you need exceeds the recommended amount, try using a more concentrated CBD oil.

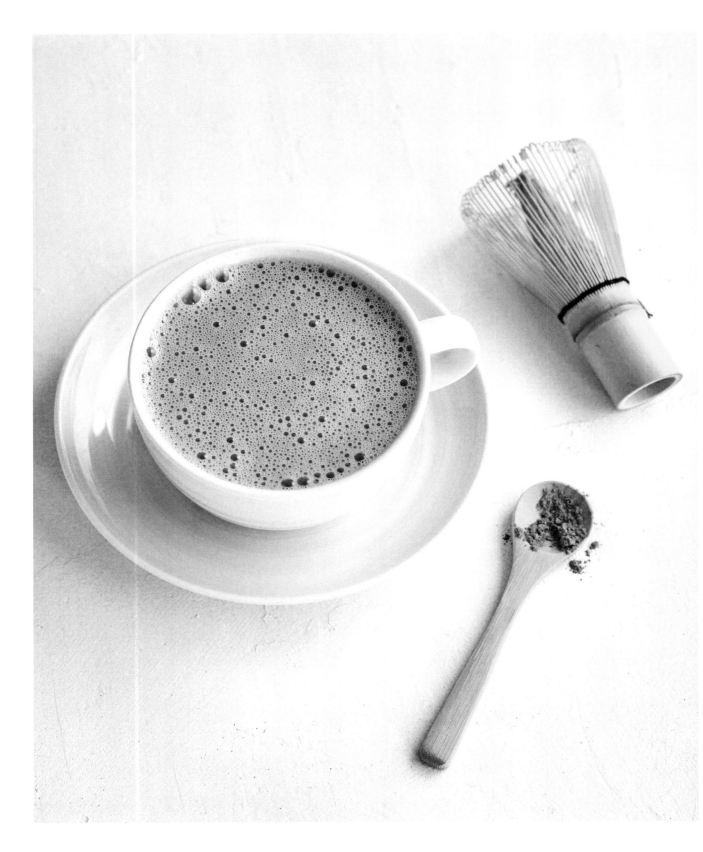

MATCHA LATTE

For a calm and focused morning, reach for this latte. Matcha delivers powerful antioxidants, as well as a caffeine boost without the crash. Smooth, creamy, and lightly sweet, it's everything you need.

TIME: 10–15 MINUTES	MAKES: 2 CUPS (480ML)	SERVES: 2

1 cup (240ml) nondairy milk
2 servings of CBD oil, but no more than 1 tsp (5ml) total
1 cup (240ml) water
2 tsp (5g) powdered matcha tea
1 tsp sugar or other sweetener

1. In a small saucepan, combine the nondairy milk and CBD oil. Place over medium-low heat and gently heat until warm but not boiling. Set aside.

2. In a small saucepan or kettle, heat the water to 170–180°F (77–82°C). (Do not exceed 180°F [82°C] or the tea will be very bitter.) While the water heats, prepare two cups with 1 tsp matcha tea and ½ tsp sugar in each cup.

3. Pour the hot water into the cups with the tea and sugar. Whisk. Add ½ cup (120ml) CBD-infused milk to each cup and whisk again. Serve immediately.

BIRTHDAY CAKE BHANG

This creamy, cake-inspired take on the traditional bhang beverage is infused with CBD and the dreamy flavor of orange flower water. Lightly sweet and delicately floral, it's sure to soothe.

TIME: 20 MINUTES   MAKES: 2 CUPS (480ML)   SERVES: 2

½ cup (120ml) half and half
1 cup (240ml) whole milk
1½ tbsp (15g) sugar or
  other sweetener
2 tsp (10ml) vanilla extract
2 servings of CBD oil, but no
  more than 2 tsp (10ml) total
1 tbsp (15ml) orange
  flower water
orange zest, to garnish

1. In a small saucepan, heat the half and half, milk, sugar or sweetener, and vanilla over medium heat. Stir continuously until hot and steaming, but not boiling. Add the CBD oil and whisk thoroughly.

2. Remove from the heat and add the orange flower water. Whisk again and pour into cups. Sprinkle orange zest over top to garnish. Serve immediately.

OH, VIENNA!

Whipped cream infused with CBD and a kiss of vanilla makes a sweet, creamy topping for this Viennese-style coffee. If you're not a coffee drinker, try it on hot cocoa or your favorite fresh fruits.

TIME: 5 MINUTES, PLUS 15 MINUTES TO BREW COFFEE	MAKES: 3 CUPS (710ML)	SERVES: 4

½ cup (120ml) heavy whipping cream
2 tsp (8g) sugar
1 tsp (5ml) vanilla extract
4 servings of CBD oil, but no more than 2 tsp (10ml) total
3 cups (710ml) freshly brewed hot coffee
ground cinnamon, to garnish

1. In a large bowl or the bowl of a stand mixer, combine the cream, sugar, vanilla, and CBD oil. Using a mixer with a wire whisk attachment, beat on high speed until the cream forms soft peaks.

2. Pour the hot coffee into 4 small cups, leaving a little space at the top of each cup. Add a large dollop of whipped cream to each cup, sprinkle with cinnamon, and serve immediately.

TIP:
The CBD-infused whipped cream can also be prepared in a whipped cream maker. Combine the cream, sugar, vanilla, and CBD oil, and follow the manufacturer's instructions.

TUMMY TEA

This fresh and very potent ginger decoction is the gateway to relief for an upset stomach. The combination of CBD, fresh ginger root, and spearmint will aid digestion and soothe nausea.

TIME: 20 MINUTES	MAKES: 2 CUPS (500ML)	SERVES: 2

2½ cups (590ml) water
3 thumb-sized pieces of ginger root, finely chopped (more if you like a strong ginger flavor)
2 sprigs of fresh spearmint
2 tbsp (30ml) whole milk
2 servings of CBD oil, but no more than 1 tsp (5ml) total
2 tsp honey or other sweetener

1. In a small saucepan, combine the water, chopped ginger, and mint. Place over medium heat and bring to a simmer. Cover and simmer for 15 minutes.

2. While the ginger and mint are simmering, warm the milk and CBD oil gently in a small saucepan over low heat or in the microwave for 30 seconds. Whisk thoroughly to combine.

3. Remove the ginger and mint water from the heat and strain the liquid into individual cups for serving. Discard the solids.

4. Add the warm milk and CBD mixture in even amounts to each cup. Add ½ tsp honey to each cup and whisk thoroughly. Serve immediately.

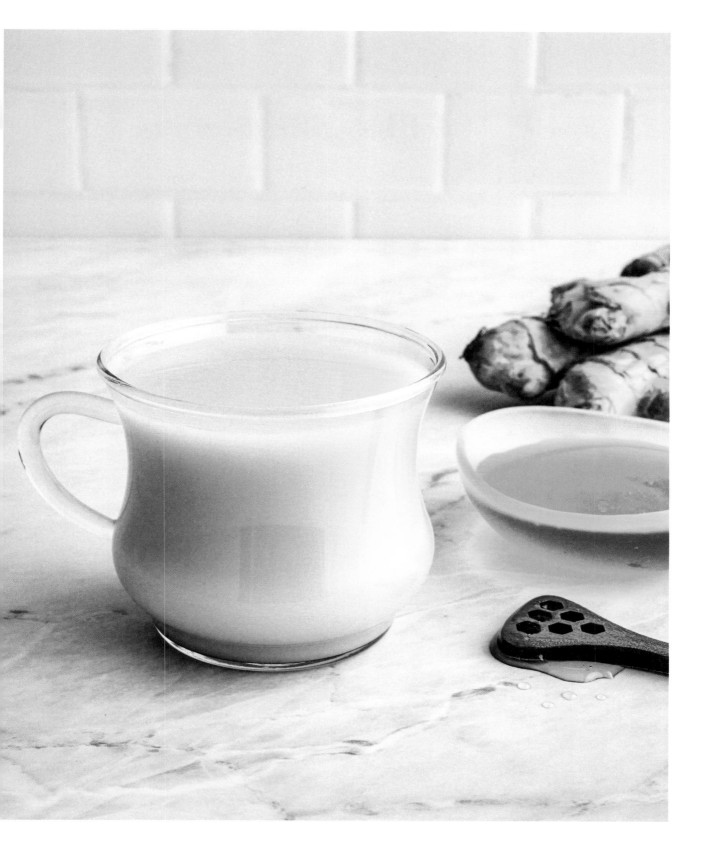

DESERT BLOSSOM COFFEE

This traditional beverage is an energizing afternoon pick-me-up infused with CBD and the spicy, floral flavors of cardamom and rose water. Use finely ground Turkish- or Arabic-style coffee, and serve in small espresso cups.

TIME: 10–15 MINUTES	MAKES: 1 CUP (237ML)	SERVES: 2–3

1 cardamom pod
3 tbsp (45ml) whole milk
2–3 servings of CBD oil, but no more than 1 tsp (5ml) total
¾ cup (180ml) water
2 tbsp (12g) finely ground whole-bean medium to dark roast coffee (not instant coffee)
¼–½ (1–2ml) tsp rose water
honey or other sweetener, to taste

1. With a mortar and pestle, break open the cardamom pod and remove the seeds. Crush the cardamom seeds to release the flavor. (Discard the pod.)

2. In a small saucepan on the stove, or in a cup in the microwave, gently heat the milk and then stir the CBD oil into it. Transfer to a small pitcher for service with the coffee.

3. In a saucepan, whisk together the water, coffee, and crushed cardamom seeds. Place over medium heat until it comes to a boil. Remove from heat. Add a splash of rose water to the pan, and whisk until slightly foamy on top.

4. Pour into espresso cups and serve immediately with the CBD-infused milk and your preferred sweetener on the side.

A BULLETPROOF MORNING

Bulletproof coffee features grass-fed butter or ghee for added healthy fats. This CBD-infused version can be made with any hot, freshly brewed coffee. Try it with flavored coffee beans like vanilla or chocolate almond for extra flavor.

TIME: 5 MINUTES	MAKES: 2 CUPS (480ML)	SERVES: 2

2 cups (480 ml) freshly brewed
  hot coffee
1 tbsp (15ml) grass-fed ghee
2 servings of CBD oil, but no
  more than 1 tsp (5ml) total
sugar or other sweetener,
  to taste

1. In a blender, combine the hot brewed coffee, grass-fed ghee, CBD oil, and sweetener. Blend on high for 1–2 minutes or until frothy.

2. Pour into coffee cups and serve immediately with sweetener, if desired.

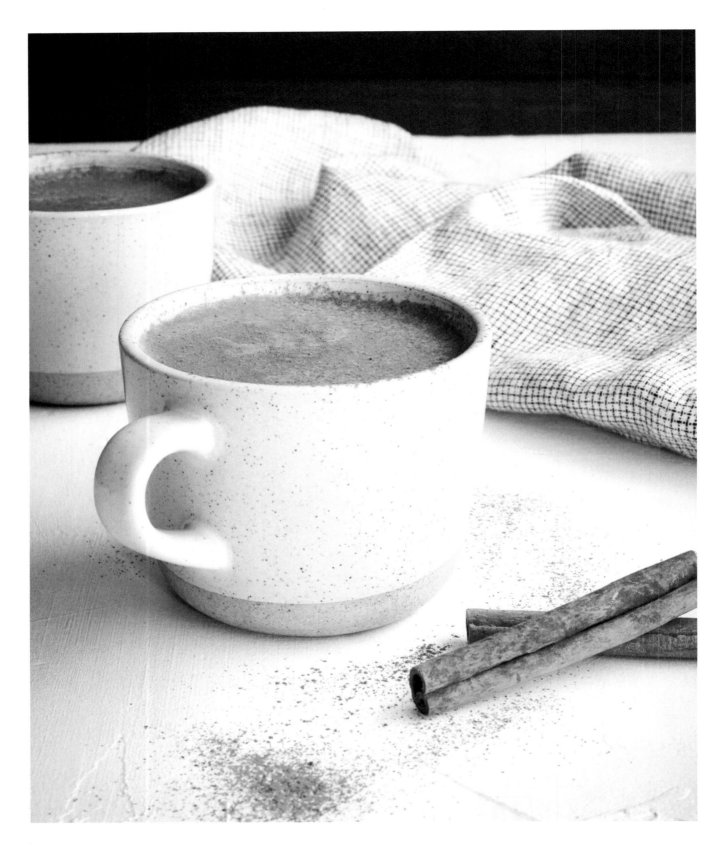

MEXICAN HOT CHOCOLATE

An invigorating and nourishing hot cocoa beverage infused with CBD and the flavor of true cinnamon, with a dash of heat from cayenne. Use Ceylon cinnamon to give this hot cocoa a distinctive sweet and floral cinnamon flavor.

TIME: 15 MINUTES	MAKES: 2 CUPS (480ML)	SERVES: 2

2 cups (480ml) whole milk
2 tbsp (6g) cocoa powder
1 tbsp (4g) sugar or other sweetener
½ tsp (1g) ground cinnamon, preferably Ceylon
1 tsp (5ml) vanilla extract
dash of cayenne
2–3 servings of CBD oil, but no more than 1 tsp (5ml) total
2 cinnamon sticks, to garnish

1. In a small saucepan, whisk together the milk, cocoa powder, sugar, cinnamon, vanilla, and cayenne. Heat over medium to medium-high heat until the mixture is hot but not boiling, and the sugar and cocoa powder are fully incorporated. Whisk frequently to prevent scorching.

2. Remove from the heat and whisk in the CBD oil before pouring into cups. Serve immediately with a cinnamon stick to garnish and enhance flavor.

GOLDEN MILK

A creamy and mildly spicy comfort beverage infused with CBD oil to bring relief at any time of the day. Fresh turmeric root lends a brighter, fresher flavor than powdered turmeric, and black peppercorns aid the bioavailability of the turmeric.

TIME: 20 MINUTES	MAKES: 2 CUPS (480ML)	SERVES: 2

2 cups (480ml) whole milk
2 thumb-sized fresh turmeric roots, coarsely chopped
6 whole black peppercorns
2 servings of CBD oil but no more than 1 tsp (5ml) total
honey or other sweetener, to taste

1. In a small saucepan, combine the milk, chopped turmeric roots, and black peppercorns. Place over medium-low heat and bring to a simmer. Simmer for 15 minutes, whisking frequently. Take care not to let the mixture boil so the milk doesn't scald.

2. Strain the turmeric and peppercorns from the milk and then pour immediately into cups for serving. Add one serving of CBD oil per cup and whisk to emulsify the oil into the hot golden milk. Sweeten as desired and top with a sprinkle of freshly-ground black pepper before serving.

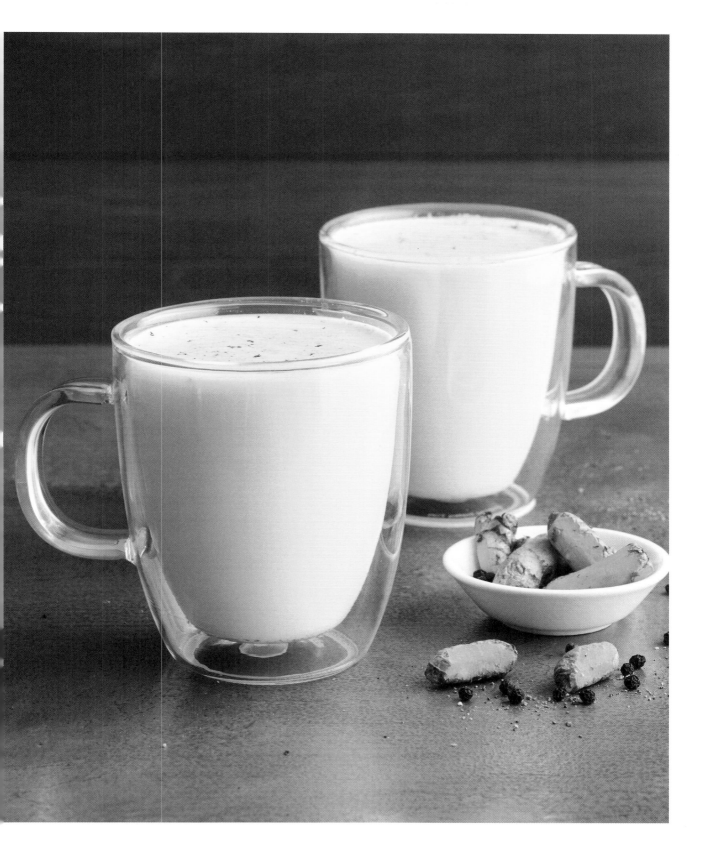

PUNJABI CHAI

This is a CBD-infused twist on the traditional tea beverage from the Punjab region, which uses milk instead of water to brew black tea with spices. Sweeten with jaggery or brown sugar cubes for the most authentic flavor experience.

TIME: 10 MINUTES	MAKES: 2 CUPS (500ML)	SERVES: 2

2¼ cups (540ml) whole milk
1 tbsp (4g) loose leaf Assam or
 black tea
5 clove buds
1 star anise pod
1 cinnamon stick
2 cardamom pods, seeds only
2 servings of CBD oil, but no
 more than 1 tsp (5ml) total
jaggery sugar or other
 sweetener, as desired

1. In a small saucepan, combine the milk, tea leaves, cloves, star anise, cinnamon stick, and cardamom seeds. Heat on medium-low until a simmer is reached. Simmer for 3 minutes, whisking frequently. Take care not to let the mixture boil so that the milk doesn't scald.

2. Strain the tea leaves and whole spices from the milk and pour immediately into cups for serving. Add one serving of CBD oil per cup and stir to emulsify the oil into the hot tea–infused milk. Sweeten as desired, and serve.

SALTED CARAMEL CRÈME

The much-loved flavor of salted caramel makes this creamy dessert beverage irresistibly delicious. The rich flavor is reminiscent of crème brûlée, and it is best served in small espresso cups.

TIME: 15 MINUTES	MAKES: 1½ CUPS (360ML)	SERVES: 2

1½ cups (360ml) half and half
2 tbsp (38g) turbinado sugar or brown sugar
½ tsp (2g) sea salt
2 tsp (10ml) vanilla extract
2 servings of CBD oil, but no more than 2 tsp (10ml) total

1. In a small saucepan, combine the half and half, sugar, salt, and vanilla. Place over medium heat and stir continuously until the sugar fully dissolves and the mixture is steaming and begins a light simmer. Add the CBD oil and whisk vigorously.

2. Remove from the heat. Pour into cups and serve immediately.

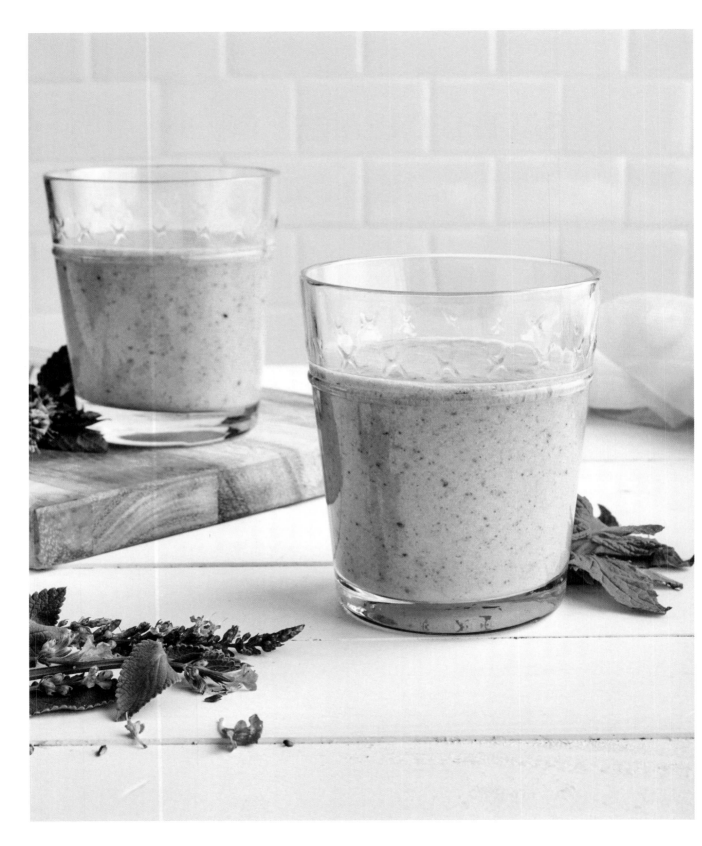

FRESH GREEN SMOOTHIE

Filling and nutritious, this green smoothie features a sweet, creamy base of coconut and banana balanced by the tart flavors of kiwi and green apple. Spinach and protein powder lend a nutritional boost.

TIME: 10 MINUTES	MAKES: 3 CUPS (710ML)	SERVES: 2

2 cups (480ml) coconut milk

2 servings of CBD oil but no more than 1 tsp (5ml) total

1 scoop plain or vanilla protein powder

3 medium kiwi, peeled

1 cup (30g) baby spinach

4–5 fresh mint leaves

2 medium green apples, cored, but not peeled

1 large banana

1 cup (240ml) ice chips

1. In a blender, combine the coconut milk and CBD oil. Blend until smooth and thoroughly combined.

2. Add the protein powder, kiwi, spinach, mint leaves, green apples, banana, and ice chips. Blend until smooth and creamy. Pour into two glasses, and serve immediately.

TIP:
For a colder smoothie, chill all of the ingredients except for the CBD oil and the banana in the fridge until very cold before making this recipe.

ROSEBERRY SMOOTHIE

A floral and sweet berry smoothie that will delight your senses—with no added sugar or other sweetener. The cooling properties of rose water paired with CBD make a soothing, refreshing beverage.

TIME: 3 MINUTES	MAKES: 2–3 CUPS (570-810ML)	SERVES: 2

1–2 cups (240–480ml) almond milk
2 cups (500g) mixed frozen berries such as strawberry, blueberry, or raspberry
1 tbsp (15ml) culinary rose water
2 servings of CBD oil, but no more than 1 tsp (5ml) total
2 tsp (10ml) orange juice or 1 tsp (5ml) lemon juice
rose petals, to garnish
fresh raspberries, to garnish

1. Place all ingredients, except garnishes, in a blender, starting with 1 cup (240ml) almond milk. Blend on high for 2 minutes or more to create a smooth and creamy beverage, adding additional almond milk as needed to achieve your desired consistency.

2. Pour into glasses and garnish with fresh or dried rose petals and a few fresh raspberries before serving.

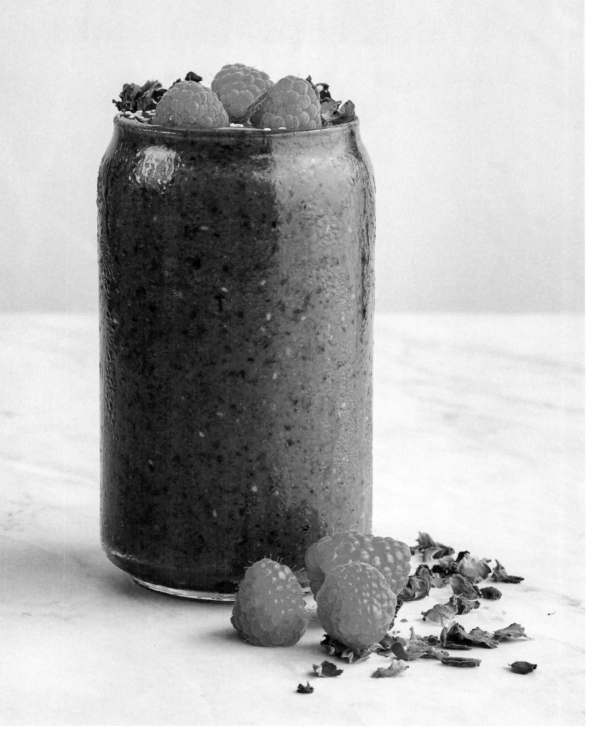

CHERRY LIMEADE SMOOTHIE

*A CBD-infused twist on the classic flavor combination of cherry and
lime, this effervescent smoothie is the perfect refresher for muscle pain.
Enjoy ice-cold. Frozen cherries, pre-pitted, work best in this recipe.*

TIME: 5 MINUTES, PLUS 3 HOURS TO SOAK	MAKES: 3 CUPS (710ML)	SERVES: 2

½ cup (120g) raw cashews
1½ cups (360ml) cold, sparkling water
2 servings of CBD oil, but no more than 1 tsp (5ml) total
1½ cups (200g) frozen, pitted cherries
juice of 1 lime
honey or other sweetener, to taste

1. Place the cashews in a medium bowl. Add water to cover cashews by at least 1 inch (2.5cm) and let soak for at least 3 hours. Drain.

2. In a blender, combine the sparkling water, soaked cashews, and CBD oil and blend thoroughly until milklike and frothy.

3. Add the frozen cherries and lime juice, and blend again until smooth. Taste and add sweetener if desired, and blend to combine. Serve immediately in chilled glasses.

ISLAND AFTERNOON SMOOTHIE

Coconut, pineapple, banana, and mango lend their tropical flavors to this creamy smoothie. High in protein and nutritious fats, it makes a satisfying meal and can serve as a meal-replacement shake.

TIME: 5 MINUTES	MAKES: 3 CUPS (710ML)	SERVES: 2

2 cups (480ml) coconut milk
2 cups (410g) cubed pineapple
1 medium banana
1 medium mango, sliced
2 scoops vanilla protein powder
1 cup (240ml) crushed ice
2 servings of CBD oil, but no
  more than 1 tsp (5ml) total
2 slices of fresh pineapple,
  to garnish

1. Place all ingredients in a blender. Blend on high for 2 minutes or more to create a smooth and creamy beverage.

2. Pour into glasses and garnish with a fresh pineapple slice.

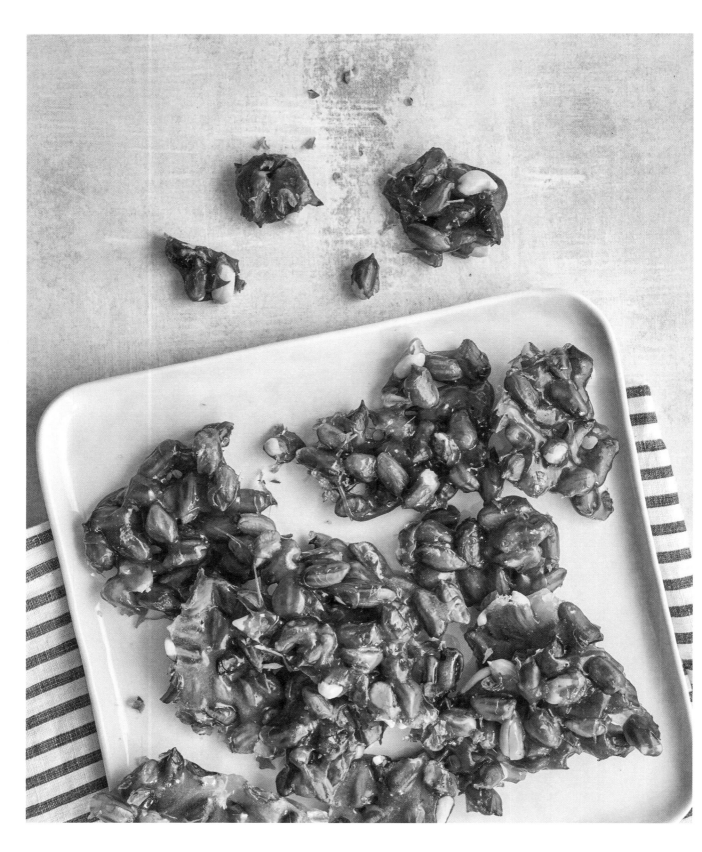

WILD PEANUT BRITTLE

The jungle peanut is a wild superfood that grows in Brazil and is not genetically modified like many commercially grown peanuts. It makes an amazing peanut brittle—especially when infused with CBD.

TIME: 35 MINUTES, PLUS 20 MINUTES TO COOL	MAKES: 12OZ (340G)	SERVES: 6–8 SERVINGS

1 cup (100g) turbinado or jaggery sugar
½ cup (120ml) water
1 tsp (5ml) vanilla extract
½ (1g) tsp salt
2 tbsp (30ml) ghee
6–8 servings of CBD oil, but no more than 2 tsp (10ml) total
½ tsp (1g) baking powder
1–1½ cups (165g) raw wild jungle peanuts

1. In a small saucepan, combine the sugar, water, vanilla, and salt. Heat over medium-low heat, stirring until sugar is dissolved.

2. Clip a candy thermometer to the pan and continue to cook on medium-low until the sugar mixture reaches 300°F (149°C), about 30 minutes. Turn off the heat immediately and remove from the stove.

3. Add the ghee, CBD oil, and baking powder to the sugar mixture and stir. Finally, add the peanuts, and fold these in quickly.

4. On a work surface (or baking sheet) that has been lined with parchment, turn out the mixture and spread evenly. Allow it to harden.

5. Break the brittle into the serving size you desire and store any leftovers in an airtight container. Consume within 1 month for best flavor.

SOOTHING HERBAL ICE POPS

Creamy coconut milk is paired with cooling mint and lavender and infused with CBD for a refreshing freezer pop that's a perfect remedy for anxiety. Try this pop any time you need to feel calm and relaxed.

TIME: 5 MINUTES, PLUS 3 HOURS TO FREEZE	MAKES: 4 ⅓-CUP (80ML) POPS	SERVES: 4

1 cup (106g) powdered coconut milk
½ cup (120ml) very hot tap water
1 tbsp (15ml) lemon juice
½ tsp (.5g) dried lavender flowers
4–6 fresh mint leaves
¼ cup (60ml) agave syrup
4 servings of CBD oil, but no more than 2 tsp (10ml) total

1. In a blender, combine all of the ingredients and blend until smooth and creamy, about 4 minutes.

2. Pour into ice pop molds and insert the sticks. Place in the freezer for at least 3 hours or until fully frozen. Consume within 1 month for best flavor.

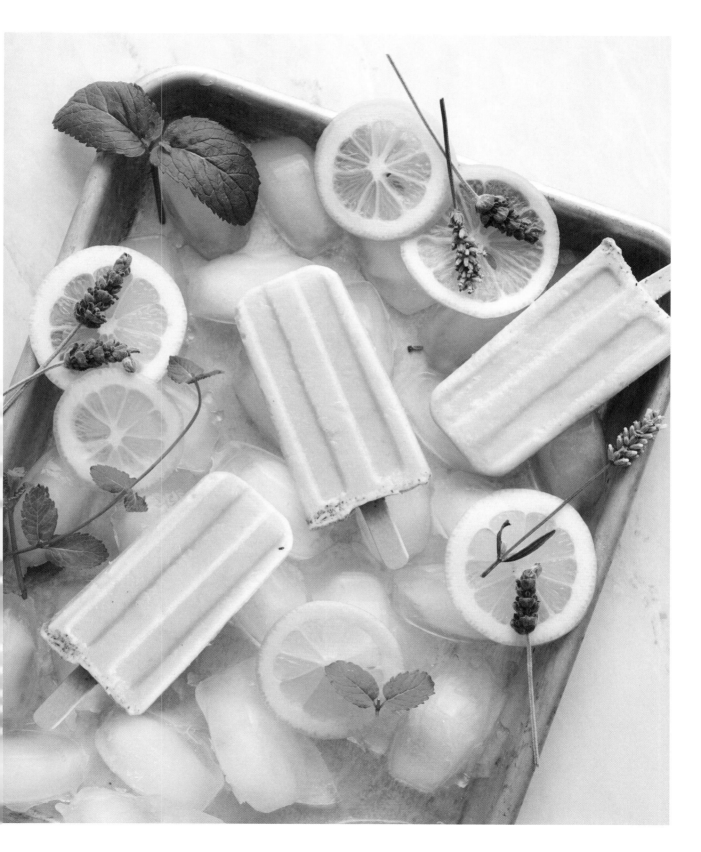

BEAR HUGS

These gummies offer a sweet little hug when you need one. Blood orange juice gives them a deep red color, but any freshly squeezed juice can be used. Use a bear-shaped silicone candy mold for a traditional gummy bear shape.

TIME: 30 MINUTES, PLUS 30 MINUTES TO SET	MAKES: 48 MINI GUMMY BEARS	SERVES: 4–6

1 cup (240ml) freshly squeezed blood orange juice or other freshly squeezed juice

4 tsp (26g) sugar

5 tbsp (37g) agar agar

4–6 servings of CBD oil, but no more than ½ tsp (2.5ml) total

1. In a small saucepan, bring the juice to a boil over medium heat, and cook until it reduces to about ⅔ cup (160ml). Add the sugar, stir to dissolve, and remove from the heat.

2. To speed cooling, pour the juice into a bowl and refrigerate until it reaches room temperature, about 20 minutes.

3. Remove the cooled juice from the refrigerator, pour it back into the saucepan, and add the agar agar a little bit at a time, stirring after each addition until it is fully dissolved.

4. Return the saucepan to the stove over medium-low heat. Add the CBD oil and stir continuously until the juice thickens to a syruplike consistency, nearly as thick as honey. Remove from the stove.

5. Working quickly, spoon the gummy mixture into the mold, or use a kitchen syringe to draw it up and inject it into the mold. Refrigerate for 30 minutes.

6. Remove from the refrigerator and pop the gummies from the mold into an airtight storage container. Store in the refrigerator and consume within 2 weeks.

TIP:
This recipe will only work with a small amount of oil. To boost the CBD in your gummies, use a concentrated form of CBD oil with a high milligram dosage.

SPICY COCOA BITES

These CBD-infused cocoa bites do not require baking and are ready in just a few minutes. With their rich chocolate flavor and pop of warming spices, they make a simple and satisfying snack.

TIME: 15 MINUTES, PLUS 20 MINUTES TO COOL	MAKES: 12 BITES	SERVES: 12

½ cup (80g) almond flour
¼ cup (40g) maca root powder
1 tbsp + 1 tsp (8g) ground ginger
¼ tsp (.5g) ground cardamom
dash of cayenne
1 tsp (5ml) vanilla extract
¼ cup (80g) sugar or coconut sugar
¼ cup (65g) cocoa powder
⅜ cup + 1 tbsp (104ml) coconut oil, softened
12 servings of CBD oil, but no more than 1 tbsp (15ml) total
powdered sugar, to coat

1. In a medium bowl, combine the almond flour, maca powder, ginger, cardamom, and cayenne. Add the vanilla and mix well. Add the sugar and cocoa and thoroughly combine. Set aside.

2. In a small bowl, stir together the softened coconut oil and the CBD oil until thoroughly combined.

3. Using a spatula, scrape the CBD-infused coconut oil into the bowl with the dry ingredients. Mix thoroughly until you have a dough that can be rolled into balls.

4. Line a plate with parchment paper. Roll the dough into 12 1½-inch (3.8-cm) balls and place on the parchment paper. Refrigerate for 20 minutes. The bites should be firm when removed from the refrigerator.

5. Prepare a small bowl with powdered sugar and roll the bites until well coated. Enjoy immediately or store in an airtight container in the refrigerator. Consume within 1 month for best flavor.

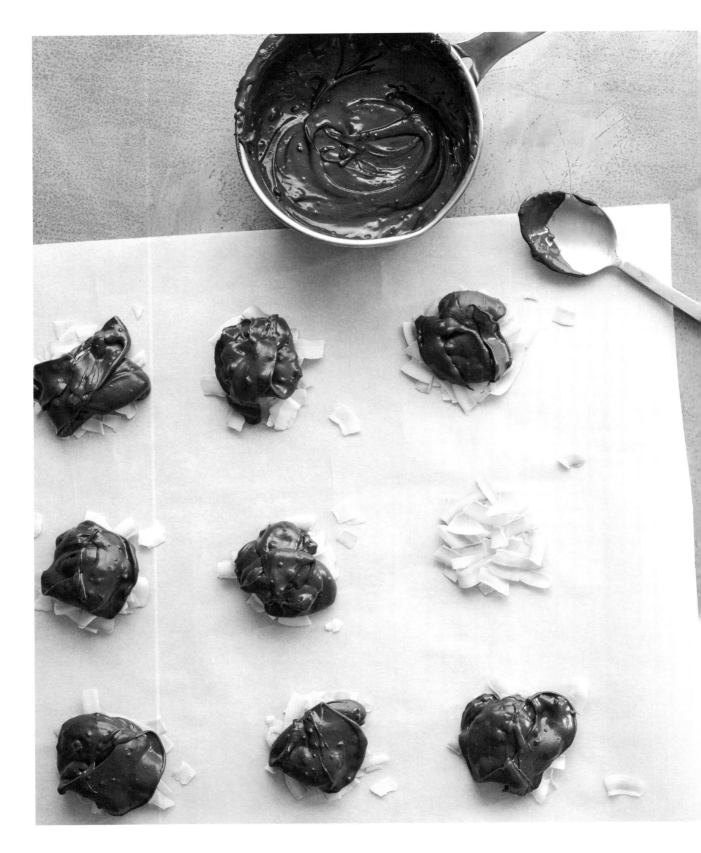

TOASTY TURTLES

The decadence of dark chocolate comes together with the benefits of CBD in a recipe that is simple to prepare in just a few minutes. Toasted coconut chips give these chocolate turtles a crisp bite and a nutty flavor.

TIME: 25 MINUTES, PLUS 30 MINUTES TO HARDEN	MAKES: 24 2-IN (5CM) TURTLES	SERVES: 12

1½ cups (75g) toasted coconut chips

1½ cups (260g) dark chocolate chips

12 servings of CBD oil, but no more than 1 tbsp (15ml) total

1. Line a baking sheet with parchment paper. On the prepared sheet, distribute the coconut chips into small piles of about 1 tbsp (2g) and in rows approximately 3 inches (7.6cm) apart to keep the candy from running together. Set aside.

2. In a double boiler over medium heat, melt the chocolate chips, stirring until fully melted. Remove from the heat and immediately stir in the CBD oil.

3. Working quickly, drizzle the melted chocolate in even amounts over the coconut chip piles until the chocolate has covered the coconut. If the melted chocolate begins to harden in the pan before you can finish, put it back in the double boiler until it melts sufficiently to drizzle over the coconut again.

4. Place the baking sheet in the refrigerator and allow to harden for 30 minutes. Once solid, transfer to an airtight container and store in a cool cabinet or in the refrigerator. Consume within 1 month for best flavor.

APRICOT CRUMBLE PIES

Tart apricots and nutty almonds come together in this lightly sweetened and gluten-free dessert. The superfood ingredient of maca powder along with almond flour makes for an especially nutritious and healthy crumble topping.

TIME: 35 MINUTES, PLUS 20 MINUTES TO COOL	MAKES: 4 5-IN (12.7CM) PIES	SERVES: 4

1¼ lb (875g) fresh, unrefrigerated apricots
1 tbsp (15ml) lemon juice
¼ cup (80g) sugar

For the topping
2 tbsp (20g) maca root powder
½ cup (80g) almond flour, packed
⅓ cup (85g) sugar
1 tsp (1.5g) ground cinnamon
¼ tsp (.5g) ground cardamom
½ tsp (2.5g) sea salt
½ tsp (2.5ml) vanilla extract
1½ tbsp (45ml) coconut oil, melted
4 servings of CBD oil, but no more than 2 tsp (10ml) total

1. Preheat the oven to 325° F (163°C). Place the apricots in a large heatproof bowl. In a pan or kettle on the stove, boil enough water to completely cover the apricots. Pour boiling water over the apricots and allow them to sit for 3–5 minutes until the skin becomes easy to pull off.

2. Drain the hot water and rinse the apricots in cool water. Remove the skins (they should slide off easily). Cut the peeled apricots into quarters and discard the pits.

3. In a medium bowl, toss the sliced apricots with the lemon juice and sugar. Set aside.

4. In a small bowl, combine the maca powder, almond flour, sugar, cinnamon, cardamom, sea salt, and vanilla. Add the coconut oil and CBD oil to the mixture and mash in to distribute evenly, creating a crumbly texture.

5. Divide the apricots evenly among 4 individual-sized pie dishes. Spoon an equal portion of the crumble mixture over the apricots in each dish.

6. Bake for 15 minutes or until lightly browned on top. Remove from the oven and allow to cool for at least 20 minutes before serving.

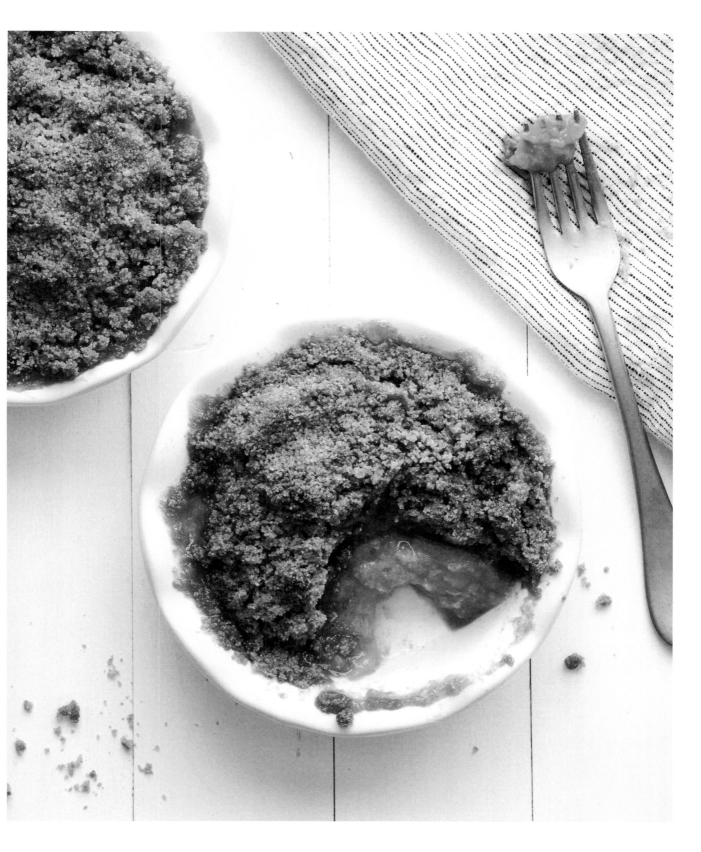

PISTACHIO-STUFFED DATES

Naturally sweet and deliciously chewy, Medjool dates are even more decadent when stuffed with a blend of spiced pistachios and CBD oil. Easily portable, they are a simple and tasty way to deliver CBD.

TIME: 15 MINUTES, PLUS 20 MINUTES TO CHILL	MAKES: 24 STUFFED DATES	SERVES: 12

½ cup (60g) shelled, roasted, and salted pistachios

1½ tbsp (22ml) coconut oil, melted

12 servings of CBD oil, but no more than ½ tbsp (7.5ml) total

1 tbsp (18g) coconut or date sugar

¼ tsp (.25g) ground cardamom

½ tsp (.5g) ground cinnamon

24 large Medjool dates

24 whole raw almonds

1. In a food processor, grind the pistachios to the texture of coarse sand.

2. In a medium bowl, combine the ground pistachios, coconut oil, and CBD oil. Add the sugar, cardamom, cinnamon, and mix well.

3. With a paring knife, slice the dates lengthwise down the middle and remove the pits (if they are not pre-split and pitted), leaving a cavity to be stuffed with the pistachio filling.

4. Pack each date with about ½ tsp of the filling and press firmly together. Press an almond on top of each date and firmly press down.

5. Refrigerate the dates for at least 20 minutes until very firm. Serve immediately, or store in a covered container in the refrigerator for up to 3 weeks for the best flavor.

TIP:
Delicious when served with hot Moroccan-style gunpowder green tea, or any tea that you prefer.

KIMCHI KALE CHIPS

Salty, spicy, and slightly sweet, these snackable kale chips deliver all the flavors of kimchi. They're a healthy and delicious way to get your dose of CBD along with the nutrients of kale.

TIME: 45 MINUTES	MAKES: 8OZ (226.7G)	SERVES: 6

2–3 bunches lacinato kale
2 tbsp (30ml) coconut oil, melted
1 tbsp (15ml) sesame oil
6 servings of CBD oil, but no more than 2 tsp (10ml) total
3 large garlic cloves, grated
3 thumb-sized pieces of fresh ginger root, grated
2 tsp (10ml) fish sauce
1 tsp (5ml) rice vinegar
2 tsp (8g) sugar
1 tsp (2g) crushed red pepper flakes
½ tsp (2.5g) salt

1. Preheat the oven to 350°F (175°C). Wash the kale leaves and pat dry. Remove the large vein and tear into large pieces. Set aside.

2. In a medium bowl, combine the coconut oil, sesame oil, CBD oil, garlic, ginger, fish sauce, vinegar, sugar, red pepper flakes, and salt. Add the kale and toss to evenly cover the leaves as much as possible. Marinate for at least 15 minutes before baking.

3. Arrange the marinated kale leaves on a baking sheet in a single layer. Evenly distribute any leftover marinade by pouring over the leaves before baking.

4. Bake for 15 minutes or until kale is crispy and a little brown around the edges. Allow to cool for 5 minutes before serving. Can be stored in an airtight container with a moisture absorbing packet for up to a week.

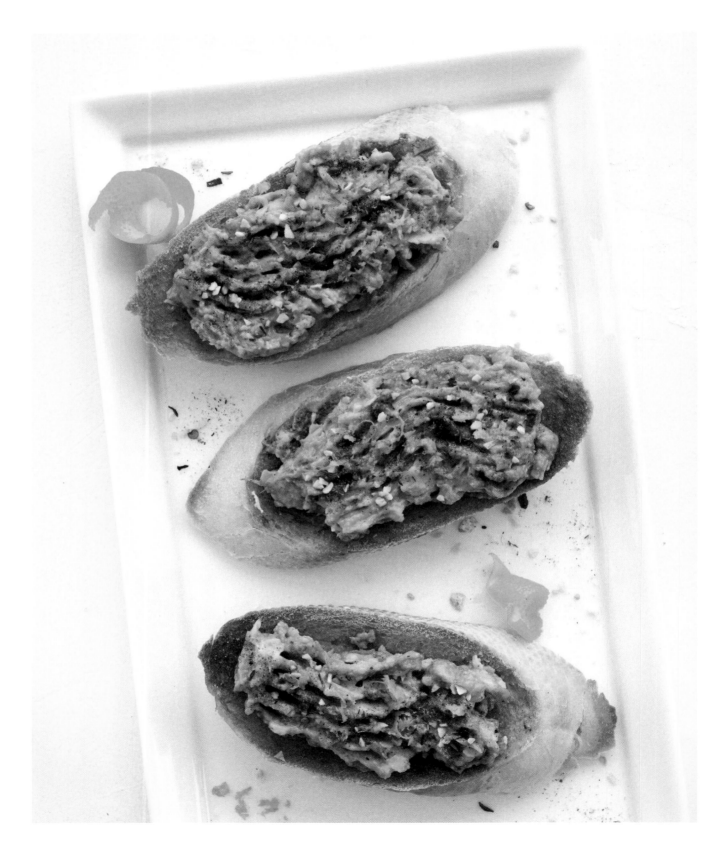

AVOCADO TOASTIES

This twist on avocado toast features Jamaican seasoning and garlic for spice and savory flavor, as well as a hint of citrus from fresh orange zest. Spread on freshly toasted baguette slices or crisp melba toast.

TIME: 10 MINUTES	MAKES: 1½ CUPS (360ML)	SERVES: 4

2 medium avocados, peeled and sliced
1 tsp (2ml) lemon juice
4 servings of CBD oil, but no more than 1½ tsp (7.5ml) total
1 tsp (4g) Jamaican jerk seasoning
½ tsp (1g) dried, minced garlic
1 tsp (1g) grated orange peel
salt, to taste
toasted bread, to serve

1. In a medium bowl, mash the avocado with the lemon juice and CBD oil. Add the Jamaican jerk seasoning, garlic, and grated orange peel, and combine thoroughly. Taste and add salt as needed.

2. To serve, spread on warm toast. Store refrigerated in an airtight container for up to 2 days.

CURRIED CARROT & CHIA CRACKERS

Chia and sunflower seeds give these gluten-free crackers an irresistible nutty crunch. Sweet carrots are complemented by bold curry spice, making them a deliciously healthy snack.

TIME: 1 HOUR 15 MINUTES

MAKES: 20–24 2-IN (5CM) CRACKERS

SERVES: 5

---

2 medium carrots
½ medium onion
1 large garlic clove
1 tbsp (15ml) lemon juice
½ cup (76g) chia seeds,
 preferably white
⅓ cup (30g) raw, shelled
 sunflower seeds
1 tbsp (15ml) basil-infused olive oil,
 or substitute 1 tbsp plain olive oil
 (15ml) and 1 tsp (2g) dried basil
5 servings of CBD oil, but no more
 than 2 tsp (10ml) total
1 tsp (1.5g) hot curry powder
½ tsp (1g) ground turmeric
½ tsp (1g) ground ginger
½ tsp (1g) sea salt, or more to taste
¼ tsp (.30g) freshly ground
 black pepper

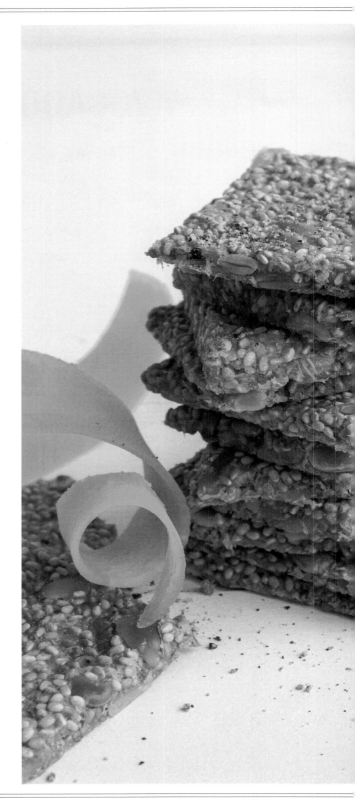

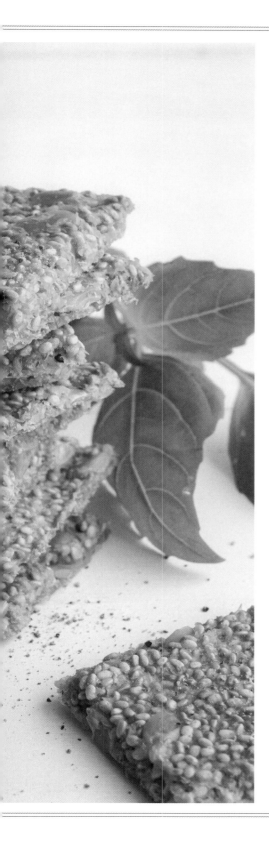

1. In a blender or food processor, combine the carrots, onion, garlic, and lemon juice. Process into a pulp.

2. Scrape the vegetable pulp into a medium bowl and mix in the chia seeds, sunflower seeds, olive oil (and basil, if using), CBD oil, curry powder, turmeric, ginger, salt, and black pepper. Combine thoroughly. Rest on the counter, covered, for at least 10 minutes.

3. Preheat the oven to 250°F (121°C) and line a baking sheet with parchment paper.

4. Spread the mixture on the baking sheet. (It should be about the thickness of a pie crust or a little thinner, depending on the thickness you prefer.) Using a fork, score the cracker dough to create about 24 2-inch (5cm) square crackers.

5. Bake for 40 minutes. Remove from the oven, turn the crackers over using a spatula, and bake for an additional 20 minutes. Depending on the humidity of your environment, the crackers may need a little more or less time in the oven. Bake and turn, and bake again until they are at the desired crispiness.

6. Cool on the counter. Store in an airtight container for up to a week for freshest flavor. If the crackers become stale from environmental humidity, pop them back in the oven at 250°F (121°C) for a few minutes to crisp.

GRASS-FED BEEF BONE BROTH

The addition of CBD oil increases the health benefits of bone broth, which is renowned for its inflammation-fighting abilities, easy-to-digest protein, and bioavailable minerals.

TIME: 10–12 HOURS

MAKES: 2QTS (2L)

SERVES: 8

3lb (1.5kg) grass-fed beef bones, mixed

2–3qt (2–3L) filtered water, enough to generously cover the bones and vegetables

1 very large yellow or white onion, cut into large pieces

3 large garlic cloves

1 tbsp (15ml) red wine vinegar

2 tsp (3g) black peppercorns

2 tsp (6g) sea salt, or more to taste

2 tsp (2g) dried marjoram

1 tsp (.5g) dried parsley

1 bay leaf

8 or more servings of CBD oil, but no more than 1 tbsp (15ml) total

1 tsp (5ml) liquid sunflower lecithin or soy lecithin

TO COOL THE BROTH FOR STORAGE:

Broth should be cooled quickly before refrigerating to avoid dangerous temperature zones at which bacteria can grow.

1. Partially fill a large bowl or pan with ice chips. Set the bowl of hot broth into the bowl with ice chips.

2. When the broth is warm to the touch, transfer it into the final containers that will go into the refrigerator. Use within 1 week or freeze.

1. Preheat the oven to 400°F (205°C). To blanch the bones before roasting, place them in a large pot and cover with water. Bring to a boil over high heat and boil for 15 minutes. Remove from the heat and discard the water.

2. On a baking sheet lined with aluminum foil, spread out the bones and roast in the oven for 20 minutes.

3. Place the roasted bones in a stock pot and add the water, onion, garlic, vinegar, peppercorns, salt, marjoram, parsley, and bay leaf. Cover and bring to a boil over high heat.

4. Lower the temperature to medium or medium-low and simmer, uncovered, for at least 1–2 hours. While simmering, skim foam at the top as you see it, and add more water, if necessary, to bring the level to at least 2 quarts (2L) and to keep the bones covered with water.

5. Cover and continue simmering for 8–10 hours. The broth is good at 8 hours, but a longer simmer will extract more protein and minerals from the bones. Remove the broth from the heat and allow it to sit while you prepare the CBD oil.

6. In a small bowl or cup, combine the CBD oil and sunflower or soy lecithin, melting together if necessary by warming in the microwave.

7. Strain the hot broth from the vegetables and bones into a large heatproof bowl. (The vegetables and bones can be discarded.)

8. Add the CBD oil and lecithin mixture to the broth and thoroughly whisk. The broth is now ready to serve. Whisk thoroughly before warming or serving again.

RAW TOMATO & RED PEPPER SOUP

A savory, CBD-infused raw soup that makes a quick and nutritious lunch. With generous servings of fresh vegetables and hemp seed, you'll have all of the protein and vitamins you need to make a complete meal.

TIME: 15 MINUTES	MAKES: 2–3 CUPS (480–710ML)	SERVES: 2

3 large or 5 medium tomatoes
1 medium red bell pepper
4 large basil leaves
1 large garlic clove
½ cup (80g) shelled hemp seed
1½ tsp (2g) dried marjoram
1 tsp (5ml) lemon juice
1 tsp (3g) sea salt
½ tsp (2g) freshly ground white pepper
¼ tsp (.25g) celery salt
2 servings of CBD oil, but no more than 1 tbsp (15ml) total
fresh basil sprigs, to garnish

1. In a blender, combine all ingredients except the fresh basil sprigs for garnish.

2. Blend on high until the soup is creamy and slightly warm, but not "cooked." It may take about 5 minutes to create a creamy and warm soup.

3. Pour into bowls and serve with a basil sprig in each bowl. Enjoy immediately.

TANDOORI TOFU LETTUCE WRAPS

Fresh and spicy, these CBD-infused, tandoori-inspired salad rolls make a nourishing main course for lunch or brunch. For a fully vegan version, use vegan mayonnaise.

TIME: 1 HOUR, PLUS 30 MINUTES TO PRESS TOFU

MAKES: 4 CUPS (900G)

SERVES: 6

1lb (455g) firm tofu
1 medium carrot, shredded
1 medium tomato, chopped
¼ cup (4g) chopped fresh
  fennel fronds
several large butter lettuce
  leaves
fresh lemon wedges, to serve

For the marinade

2 tbsp (30ml) coconut oil
6 servings of CBD oil, but no
  more than 2 tsp (10ml) total
3 tbsp (30ml) lemon juice
1 tsp (3g) curry powder
½ tsp (1g) ground ginger
1 tsp (3g) garam masala
½ tsp (1g) dried minced garlic
¼ tsp (.5g) salt

For the dressing

¾ cup (180ml) mayonnaise
2 tsp (10ml) lemon juice
½ tsp (1g) curry powder
¼ tsp (.5g) cayenne
½ tsp (1.5g) salt
¼ tsp (.5g) dried minced
  garlic
freshly ground black pepper,
  to taste

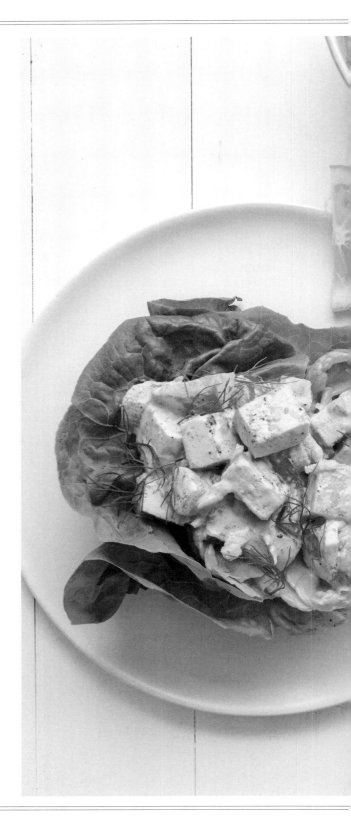

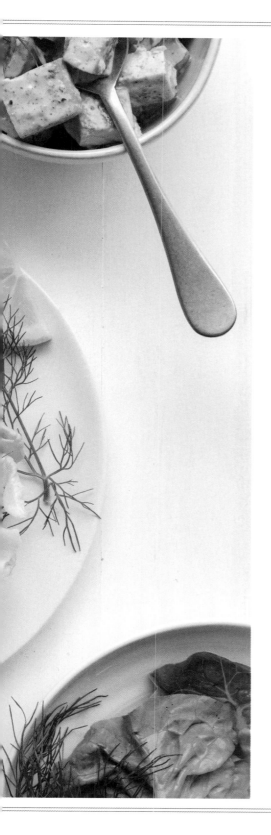

1. Press the tofu to remove excess liquid. Layer the block of tofu between two clean, folded cotton dish towels. Place a cutting board on top and then place a heavy object on the cutting board, such as a cast iron pan or small exercise weight. Let sit for at least 30 minutes. Once pressed, cut the tofu into 8 slices and set aside.

2. Preheat the oven to 375°F (190°C). In small saucepan, melt the coconut oil for the marinade over low heat. Stir in the CBD oil.

3. To make the marinade, in a medium bowl, combine the CBD-infused coconut oil, lemon juice, curry powder, ginger, garam masala, garlic, and salt. Add the tofu (it should be room temperature) and toss gently to coat. Marinate at room temperature for least 15 minutes.

4. Place the marinated tofu slices on a baking sheet and spoon all of the marinade over them. Bake for 30 minutes. Remove from the oven. Place the slices on a clean plate and allow them to cool. Cut the slices into cubes and put them in a bowl. Spoon any oil left on the baking sheet over the cubes in the bowl. Refrigerate while you prepare the dressing.

5. To make the dressing, in a medium bowl, stir together the mayonnaise, lemon juice, curry powder, cayenne, salt, garlic, and pepper (to taste).

6. Remove the tofu from the refrigerator and add the carrots, tomatoes, and fennel fronds. Toss to combine. Add the mayonnaise dressing to the tofu and vegetables and gently mix until well coated. Refrigerate for 15 minutes.

7. Arrange butter lettuce leaves on a plate, fill each one with the salad mixture, and wrap. Squeeze lemon over top and serve immediately. Refrigerate any unused portion and consume within a day for freshest flavor.

TEMPLE MASSAGE BALM

Immediate relief for headaches and muscle aches in your shoulders, neck, and back. The fresh fragrance of gingergrass comes together with the sweet and balsamic scent of frankincense frereana to enhance the soothing effects of CBD.

TIME: 5 MINUTES, PLUS 40 MINUTES TO SOLIDIFY	MAKES: 2OZ (60ML)	CONTAINER: STERILE ROUND TIN

2 tbsp (30ml) shea butter

1 tbsp (15ml) almond oil

½ oz (16g) raw, unfiltered beeswax (bar or pellet form)

1 tbsp (15ml) or less CBD oil

5 drops gingergrass essential oil

10 drops frankincense frereana essential oil (do not substitute with other varieties of frankincense essential oil)

5 drops copaiba essential oil

1. In a small saucepan, gently melt together the shea butter, almond oil, beeswax, and desired amount of CBD oil until fully combined. Remove from the heat and add the essential oils of gingergrass, frankincense, and copaiba.

2. Pour into sterile and dry salve or balm container(s) and allow to cool to room temperature.

3. Affix the lid(s) and place in the refrigerator for at least 20 minutes to fully solidify. Store the unused balm in a cool, dark area. Use within 3 months for best results.

TO USE:

Apply to the temples, forehead, back of neck, or shoulders as needed. You can carry the balm in a bag or purse, but do not expose to excessively hot temperatures.

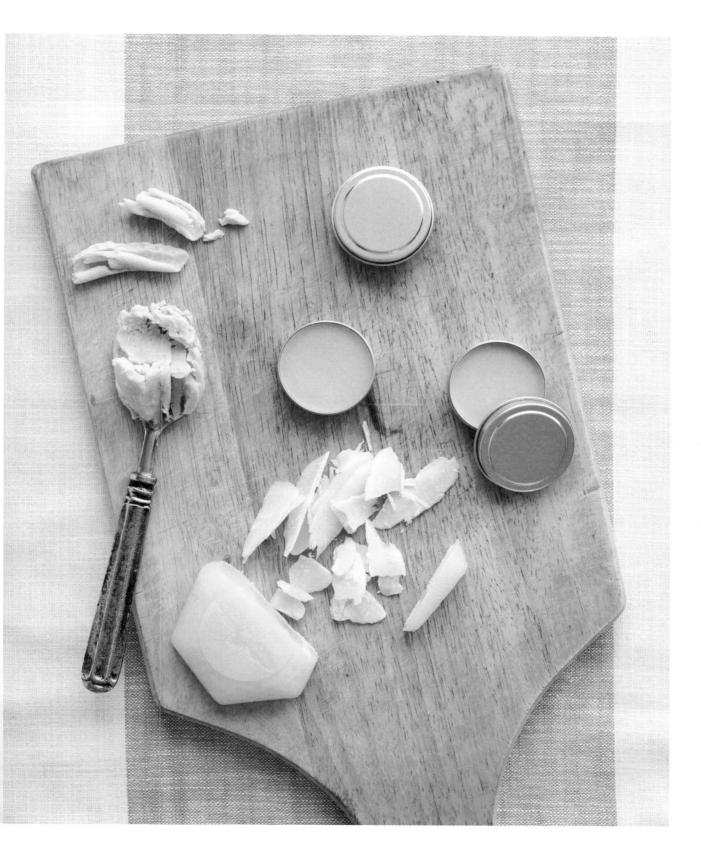

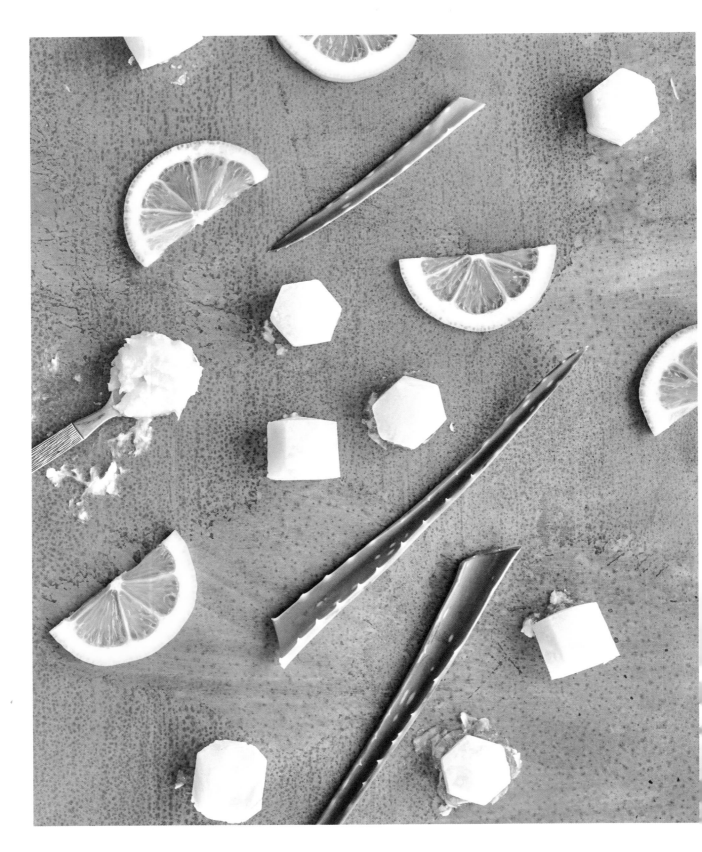

COOLING ALOE LOTION

A soothing and cooling freezer lotion infused with CBD. This lotion contains no added preservatives or fragrances, which makes it a great choice for sensitive skin. Use straight from the freezer as a convenient cube whenever you need relief.

TIME: 15 MINUTES, PLUS 2 HOURS TO FREEZE	MAKES: 10 LOTION CUBES	CONTAINER: ICE CUBE TRAY

¼ cup (60ml) coconut oil
¾ cup (180ml) preservative-free aloe vera juice, or gel from aloe vera leaves
½ tsp (2.5ml) lemon juice
2 tsp (10ml) or less CBD oil

1. In a small saucepan or microwaveable dish, warm and melt the coconut oil completely.

2. In a blender, combine the aloe vera, melted coconut oil, lemon juice, and desired amount of CBD oil. Blend until creamy and smooth.

3. Use some of the lotion immediately if desired. Pour the rest of the lotion into an ice cube tray and freeze until solid.

4. Once frozen, pop the solid lotion from the tray and store in an airtight container in the freezer. Use within 3 months.

Note:
This lotion must be used within a day if it is not refrigerated, and within 3 days if it is refrigerated and not frozen. Do not use if it has been at room temperature for more than a day or refrigerated for more than 3 days.

TO USE:

Remove a lotion cube from the freezer and rub directly on to your skin, allowing the lotion to melt and absorb. The cooling lotion can soothe minor skin irritations, rashes, and sunburn.

CLEAR SKIN TONER

*Cleanse and rejuvenate inflamed and oily skin with a CBD-infused toner
that includes witch hazel–bark tea, blue chamomile essential oil, and
real rose water to cool and refresh the skin.*

TIME: 45 MINUTES	MAKES: 12OZ (355ML)	CONTAINER: STERILE GLASS BOTTLE

1 cup (240ml) distilled water
¼ cup (20g) witch hazel bark, cut and sifted
¼ cup (60ml) 150-proof or higher food-grade alcohol
5 drops blue chamomile essential oil
10 drops rosemary antioxidant extract
1 tsp (5ml) or less CBD oil
3 tbsp (45ml) culinary rose water

1. In a small saucepan, bring the distilled water to a boil and add the witch hazel bark. Remove from the heat. Cover and steep for at least 30 minutes.

2. Using a strainer lined with cheesecloth, strain the liquid from the witch hazel bark and set aside. Discard the witch hazel bark.

3. In a sterile and dry glass bottle, combine the alcohol, blue chamomile essential oil, rosemary antioxidant, and desired amount of CBD oil. Shake thoroughly to combine. Add the witch hazel bark liquid and rose water, replace the cap, and shake thoroughly again. Keep refrigerated. Use within 3 months for best results.

TO USE:
Put a little on a cotton pad and swipe over your entire face or on problem breakout areas. It can also be used as a splash.

CBD SPA MASK

Rescue irritated, oily skin with this CBD-infused herbal and clay face mask. Desert natives of yucca root and rhassoul clay come together with CBD and essential oils to absorb oil, calm inflammation, and discourage breakouts.

TIME: 5 MINUTES	MAKES: 3½OZ (100G)	CONTAINER: STERILE GLASS JAR

¼ cup (46g) yucca root powder
¼ cup (50g) rhassoul clay powder
1 tsp (3g) benzoin resin powder
1 tsp (5ml) or less CBD oil
6 drops tea tree essential oil
10 drops lemon myrtle essential oil

1. In a small bowl, combine the powdered yucca root, rhassoul clay, and benzoin resin.

2. Add the desired amount of CBD oil along with essential oils of tea tree and lemon myrtle. Mix and mash to thoroughly distribute the oils throughout the powder.

3. Store the powdered mask in a sterile, dry glass jar with a tight-fitting lid. Can be stored in the bathroom cabinet for quick access. Use within 3 months for best results.

TO USE:

1. In a small bowl, spoon out 1 tbsp (13g) or less of the mask powder depending on how much coverage you need.

2. Add enough warm water or warm, brewed black or green tea to make a paste that can be spread over the skin using a brush or your fingers. Add the liquid a little bit at a time until you have the consistency that you want.

3. Apply to the skin and allow this to remain on the skin up to an hour for best results.

4. Rinse off with cool or warm water. Pat the skin dry and allow it to breathe for at least 15 minutes before applying cosmetics or moisturizers.

PURIFYING SALT SCRUB

This skin-beautifying and exfoliating scrub infused with CBD oil offers relief to aching legs and feet. This recipe uses coarsely ground Dead Sea salt for its unique mineral profile paired with essential oils of lemon myrtle and sage.

TIME: 25 MINUTES	MAKES: 11OZ (305G)	CONTAINER: STERILE GLASS JAR

⅓ cup (80ml) raw organic coconut oil

1 tbsp (15ml) or less CBD oil

1 cup (225g) medium-coarse ground Dead Sea salt

10 drops lemon myrtle essential oil

5 drops sage essential oil

1. In a small saucepan, combine the coconut oil and CBD oil in desired amount. Melt over medium-low heat and stir. Remove from the heat, and allow to briefly cool, but not solidify.

2. Fill a sterile, dry glass jar with the Dead Sea salt. Pour the coconut oil and CBD oil mixture into the salt, add the lemon myrtle and sage essential oils, and stir to thoroughly combine.

3. Cover with a lid and refrigerate for 15 minutes. Remove from the refrigerator. The scrub is now ready for the shelf and can be used at any time. Use this product within 3 months for best results.

TO USE:

Begin with wet, warm skin that has been softened by a shower or bath. Apply the salt scrub in a circular motion, rubbing it in until skin feels fully exfoliated. Rinse with running water. Avoid shaving or waxing before using any salt scrub.

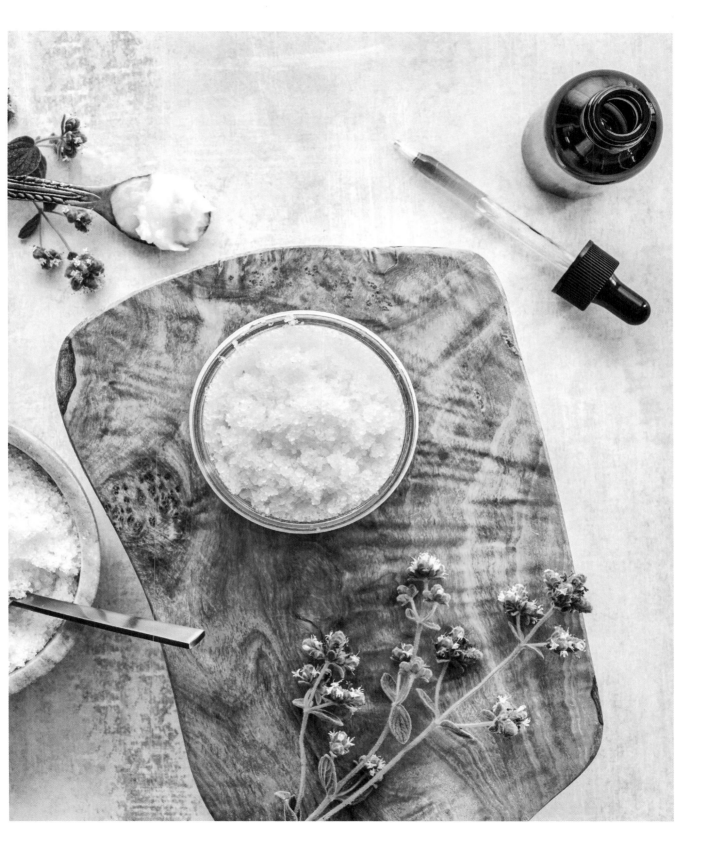

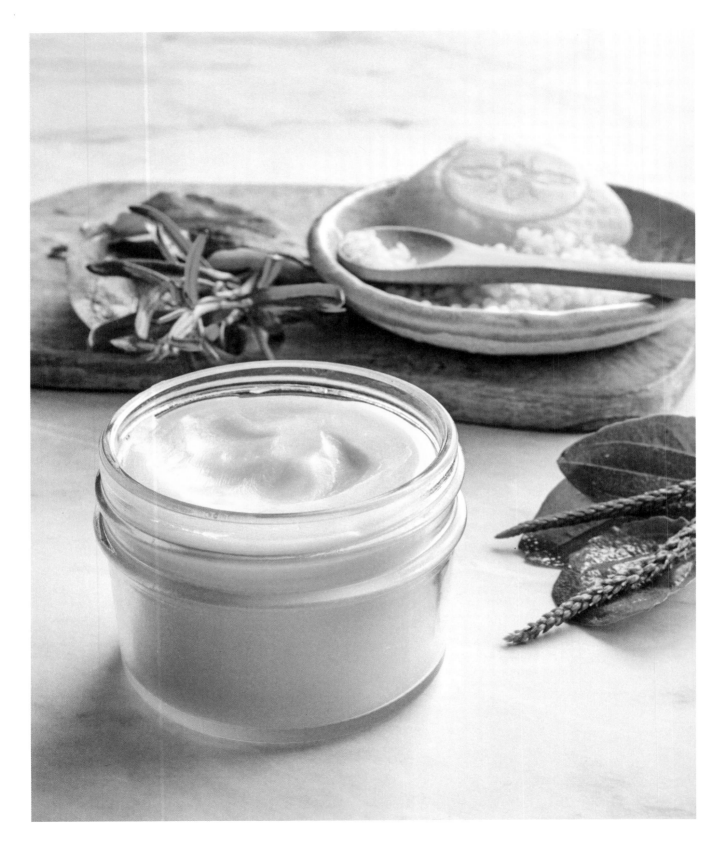

KITCHEN SINK SALVE

This salve features plantain, a common backyard weed with medicinal properties, as well as the essential oils of rosemary and myrrh to soothe and heal irritated skin. Great for everyday use and a favorite salve of many gardeners.

TIME: 1 HOUR, PLUS 1 DAY TO FORAGE AND WILT PLANTAIN	MAKES: 12OZ (360ML)	CONTAINER: STERILE GLASS JAR(S)

1 cup (20g) fresh plantain leaves
½ cup (120ml) coconut oil
¼ cup (60ml) olive oil
6.5oz (208g) raw, unfiltered beeswax (bar or pellet form)
1 tbsp (15ml) hemp seed oil
2 tsp (10ml) or less CBD oil
10 drops rosemary essential oil
20 drops myrrh essential oil

1. Forage the plantain. Pick only the leaves—you'll need at least two good bunches. Look for healthy, unblemished leaves and avoid heavily trafficked areas and lawns treated with pesticides.

2. Wash the plantain leaves thoroughly and place on a paper towel in a single layer overnight to wilt. After they have wilted, cut them into smaller pieces.

3. In a double boiler, combine the coconut oil, olive oil, and plantain and heat, stirring frequently.

4. Remove from the heat and strain the oil from the leaves. Discard the leaves. Pour the oil back into the double boiler and add the beeswax, hemp seed oil, and desired amount of CBD oil. Heat for 15 minutes.

5. Remove from the heat, add the essential oils, and stir. Pour the salve into the jar(s). Allow the jar(s) to remain on the counter and cool for 5 minutes. Affix the lids and transfer to the freezer for 30 minutes to harden.

6. Store the salve in a cool, dark place until ready to use. Use within 6 months for best results.

Note:
Plantain is one of the most common weeds in North America, and contains chemical compounds that facilitate healing and soothe irritation. Either species, *Plantago major* or *Plantago lanceolata* will work in this recipe, and both are easily found in lawns and parks.

TO USE:
Rub into dry, chapped hands to soothe and soften.

JOINT & MUSCLE SALVE

Relieve deep muscle and joint pain with the warming combination of CBD, cayenne, and essential oils. This pain-relieving salve made with beeswax, almond oil, and coconut oil absorbs quickly for fast relief anytime you need it.

TIME: 20 MINUTES, PLUS 30 MINUTES TO HARDEN	MAKES: 12OZ (365ML)	CONTAINER: STERILE GLASS JAR(S)

½ cup (120ml) almond oil
¼ cup (60ml) coconut oil
6oz (193g) raw, unfiltered beeswax (bar or pellet form)
1 tbsp (15ml) or less CBD oil
1 tsp (5ml) liquid soy or sunflower lecithin
5 drops rosemary antioxidant extract
1 tsp (1g) cayenne
10 drops ginger essential oil
6 drops black pepper essential oil
15 drops lavender essential oil

1. In a double boiler or in a saucepan over low heat, combine the almond oil, coconut oil, beeswax, desired amount of CBD oil, lecithin, rosemary antioxidant, and cayenne. Heat for 15 minutes on a low simmer or low heat until fully melted and thoroughly combined. Whisk frequently.

2. Remove from the heat. Add the essential oils of ginger, black pepper, and lavender to the salve and stir them in carefully.

3. Prepare a sterile and dry, heatproof glass jar(s). Pour the hot salve mixture into the jar(s).

4. Allow the salve to rest at room temperature for 5 minutes. Cap the salve and finish hardening in the freezer for 30 minutes. The salve is now shelf-stable and ready to use right away. Use within 3 months for best results.

TO USE:

Apply generously to sore joints and muscles. Do not apply to broken skin, get into eyes, or apply to any mucous membrane.

CBD BITTERS

CBD-infused digestive bitters made with dandelion and burdock root help to soothe over-indulgence and optimize digestion. Use as a tincture straight from the jar or vial, or serve in warm lemon-infused water.

TIME: 10 MINUTES, PLUS 2–4 WEEKS TO INFUSE	MAKES: 35 1-TSP (5ML) SERVINGS	CONTAINER: STERILE GLASS JAR OR VIAL

½ cup (130g) chopped dandelion root

¼ cup (60g) chopped burdock root

1 tbsp (4g) grated orange peel

2 tsp (5g) fenugreek seeds

2 tsp (5g) fennel seeds

¾ cup (180ml) 150-proof or higher clear liquor (rum or brandy is best)

35 servings of CBD oil, but no more than 1 tbsp (15ml) total

1. In a lidded glass jar, combine the dandelion root, burdock root, orange peel, fenugreek seeds, and fennel seeds. Stir to mix these thoroughly.

2. Pour the clear liquor over the herbs and press the herbs down so that the alcohol covers them completely. Close the jar and set in a cool, dark place for 2–4 weeks. Shake the jar once a week.

3. Decant the liquid tincture into dry, sterile glass jars or vials by straining it from the herbs using a cheesecloth-lined wire strainer. Discard solids.

4. Add the CBD oil and shake vigorously to thoroughly dissolve the oil into the alcohol tincture. Store in a dark and cool place and shake thoroughly before use.

TO USE:

Shake before using. Add 1 tsp bitters to hot lemon-infused water. Whisk thoroughly and serve with a thin lemon slice floating on top.

TENSION RELIEF ROLL-ON

Try this CBD-infused topical relief roll-on the next time you need to relieve a headache or neck tension. Featuring the soothing essential oils of lavender, spearmint, and ylang-ylang, this roll-on is perfect for day- or nighttime relief.

TIME: 12 MINUTES	MAKES: 1OZ (30ML)	CONTAINER: 2 STERILE GLASS ROLLERBALL APPLICATORS

2 tbsp (30ml) almond oil
¼ tsp (1.25ml) vitamin E oil
20 drops lavender essential oil
10 drops spearmint essential oil
5 drops ylang-ylang essential oil
2 tsp (10ml) or less CBD oil

1. In a small sterile and dry cup, combine the almond oil, vitamin E oil, essential oils, and desired amount of CBD oil. Stir to combine.

2. Fill each rollerball container with the oil mixture. Snap in the rollerball applicator and screw on the lids after filling.

3. Warm a cup of water on the stove or in the microwave and place the applicators in the hot—but not boiling—water. Allow these to warm for at least 2 minutes and then shake the applicators to evenly distribute all of the oils. Use within 6 months for best results.

TIP:
A small funnel, designed to aid in filling applicators of this size with oils, is useful for making this recipe.

TO USE:
Roll on temples, behind ears, and at the base of the neck to help relieve tension.

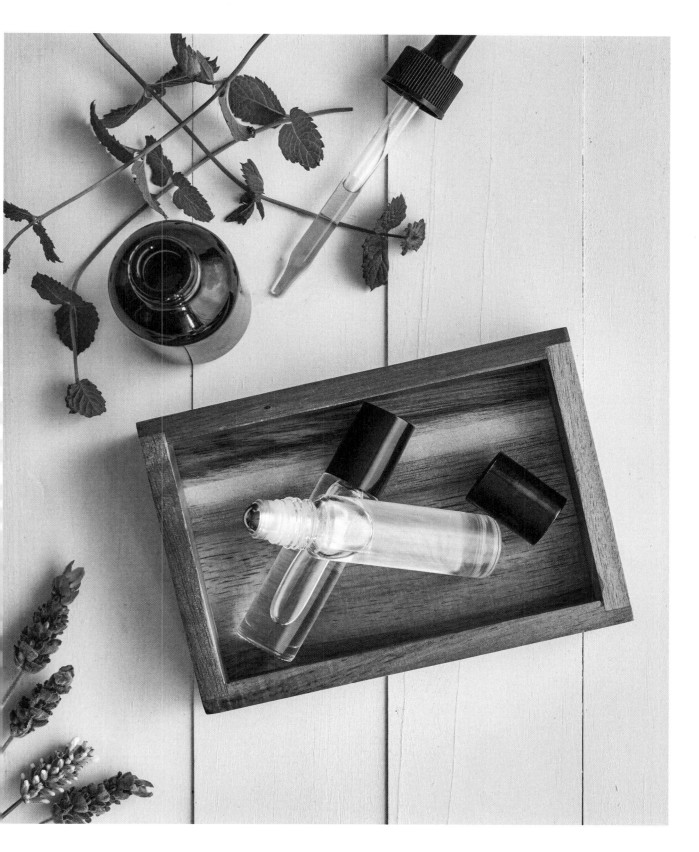

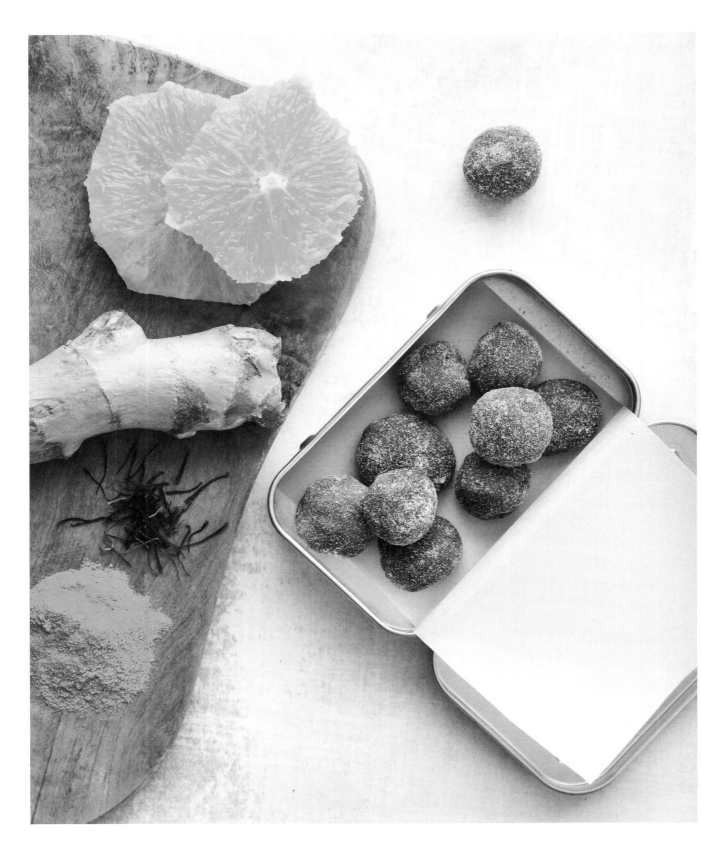

STOMACH-SOOTHING GINGER LOZENGES

Carry these lozenges for fast relief from nausea, such as motion sickness, or anytime you are feeling a bit queasy. Each lozenge delivers a serving of CBD as well as a generous dose of ginger, which has stomach-soothing properties.

TIME: 40 MINUTES, PLUS 20 MINUTES TO HARDEN	MAKES: 24 LOZENGES	SERVES: 24

¾ cup (150g) granulated sugar
¾ cup (180ml) freshly squeezed orange juice (blood oranges are preferred)
24 servings of CBD oil, but no more than 1 tbsp (15ml) total
2 tsp (4g) ground ginger

For the coating
¼ cup (31g) superfine sugar
3 tsp (6g) ground turmeric or 20 saffron threads, finely crushed

1. Prepare the coating. Combine superfine sugar and turmeric (or saffron) in a small bowl and set aside.

2. In a small saucepan, stir together the granulated sugar and orange juice. Clip a candy thermometer to the edge of the pan, and cook over low to medium-low heat. When the thermometer reaches 300°F (149°C) (hard-crack stage), immediately remove the pan from the heat.

3. After the hot sugar mixture has cooled for 1 minute, add the CBD oil and ginger, and combine thoroughly. The mixture should be similar in consistency to a thick batter.

4. Turn the mixture out on a silicone mat or parchment paper. Allow it to cool until it is warm to the touch and easy to roll between your fingers without sticking to them. Work quickly roll into ½-inch (1.27cm) balls.

5. After all of the lozenges are rolled, bury them in the superfine sugar and turmeric (or saffron) mixture and generously coat them.

6. Remove lozenges from the sugar mixture and place on a silicone- or parchment-lined baking sheet to harden in the refrigerator for 20 minutes. Store the lozenges in an airtight container and use within 2 months.

HEADACHE PASTILLES

In this herbal pastille, CBD is combined with clove and boswellia to provide quick relief for most headaches. Clove has been a go-to for pain relief for centuries across many cultures and contains terpenes that are also found in the cannabis plant.

TIME: 40 MINUTES, PLUS 20 MINUTES TO HARDEN

MAKES: 24 PASTILLES

SERVES: 24

½ cup (120ml) honey
½ cup (120ml) lemon juice
½ vanilla bean
24 serving sizes of CBD oil, but
  no more than 2 tsp (10ml) total
1 tsp (4g) Boswellia serrata
  (Indian frankincense) powder,
  fine and free of chunks
3 drops clove essential oil

For the coating
¼ cup (31g) superfine sugar
2 tsp (4g) ground turmeric

1. Prepare the coating. Combine superfine sugar and turmeric in a small bowl and set aside.

2. In a small saucepan, combine the honey and lemon juice. Slice the vanilla bean in half lengthwise and scrape the seeds from the pod using the tip of a knife. Add the scraped vanilla paste to the pan, and stir to combine thoroughly.

3. Clip a candy thermometer to the side of the pan and cook over medium-low heat. When the thermometer reading reaches 300°F (149°C) (hard-crack stage), immediately remove the pan from the heat.

4. After the hot honey mixture has cooled for 1 minute, add the CBD oil, boswellia powder, and clove essential oil and combine thoroughly. The mixture should be about the consistency of a thick batter.

5. Turn the mixture out on to a silicone mat or parchment paper and allow it to cool until it is warm to the touch and easy to roll between your fingers without sticking to them. Working quickly, roll into ½-inch (1.27cm) balls or lozenges.

6. After all of the pastilles are rolled, bury them in the sugar and turmeric mixture and generously coat them.

7. Remove from the sugar and turmeric and place on a silicone- or parchment-lined baking sheet. Allow them to harden in the refrigerator for 20 minutes.

8. Store the pastilles in an airtight container in a cool cabinet. Use within 2 months.

CHERRY BARK & ELDERBERRY LOZENGES

Chase away seasonal bugs or soothe irritated throats and coughs with this CBD-infused lozenge. Great for when you need an elderberry immune-system boost.

TIME: 40 MINUTES, PLUS 20 MINUTES TO HARDEN

MAKES: 30 LOZENGES

SERVES: 30

¼ cup (65g) superfine sugar,
 to coat
1 tbsp (6g) wild cherry bark,
 cut and sifted
3 cups (710ml) water
1 cup (250g) granulated sugar
3 tbsp (45ml) concentrated
 elderberry extract or juice
30 servings of CBD oil, but no
 more than 1 tbsp (15ml) total

1. Place the superfine sugar in a small bowl and set aside. Rinse the dried cherry bark in cool water to clean any dirt or dust. Discard the rinse water.

2. In a small saucepan, combine the rinsed cherry bark and the water. Bring to a boil over medium-high heat and continue boiling until the water reduces to 2 cups (480ml).

3. Strain the liquid from the bark and discard the bark. Return the liquid to the pan and add the granulated sugar and elderberry juice. Stir until the sugar is dissolved.

4. Clip a candy thermometer to the edge of the pan, and place over medium heat. Stir continuously until the thermometer reaches 300°F (149°C) (hard crack stage). Immediately remove from the heat.

5. After the hot sugar mixture has cooled for 1 minute, add the CBD oil and combine thoroughly. The mixture should be similar in consistency to a thick batter.

6. Turn the mixture out on a silicone mat or parchment paper and allow it to cool until it is warm to the touch and easy to roll between your fingers without sticking to them. Work quickly once the mixture has reached the warm stage and roll into 30 1-inch (2.5cm) balls or lozenges.

7. After all of the cough drops are formed, roll them in the superfine sugar until thoroughly coated. Place the cough drops on a silicone- or parchment-lined baking sheet and transfer to the refrigerator for 20 minutes to fully cool and harden.

8. Store the lozenges in an airtight container in a cool cabinet. Use within 3 months.

VANILLA MINT LIP BALM

Treat yourself to fast relief of chapped or irritated lips—and a satisfying way to enjoy a little bit of CBD with each application. Flavored with sweet vanilla and cooling mint, this soothing balm glides on easily for soft, smooth lips.

TIME: 1 HOUR, PLUS 30 MINUTES TO COOL	MAKES: 2½ OZ (75ML)	CONTAINER: 2–4 STERILE SLIDE-TOP TINS OR LIP BALM TUBES

1½oz (49g) raw, filtered beeswax (bar or pellet form)
1 tbsp (15ml) coconut oil
1 tbsp (15ml) rice bran oil
½ vanilla bean
1 tsp (5ml) or less CBD oil
¼ tsp (1.25ml) vitamin E oil
2–3 drops peppermint essential oil

1. In a small double boiler, combine the beeswax, coconut oil, and rice bran oil. Place over medium heat until melted. Add vanilla bean and process over low heat for up to 1 hour. (Longer processing will result in more intense flavor.)

2. Remove the vanilla bean from the oil and discard. Add the CBD oil, vitamin E oil, and peppermint essential oil, and thoroughly combine. Pour into lip balm containers immediately.

3. Allow the containers to rest at room temperature for 2 minutes. Cap and then place them in the freezer for 30 minutes to harden completely. The lip balm is now shelf-stable. Use within 6 months for best results.

TO USE:
Apply to the lips as you would any other lip balm, and as often as you prefer.

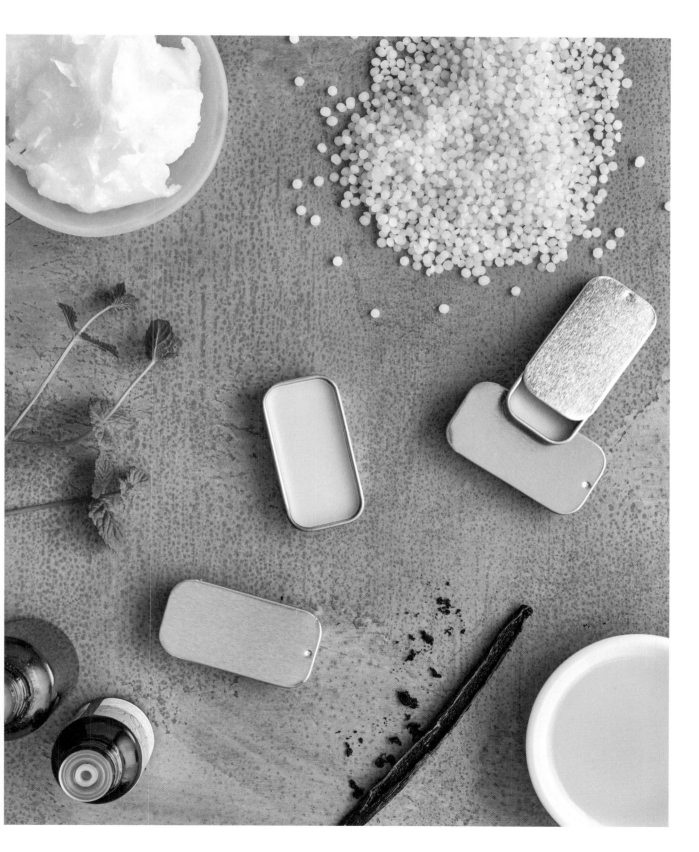

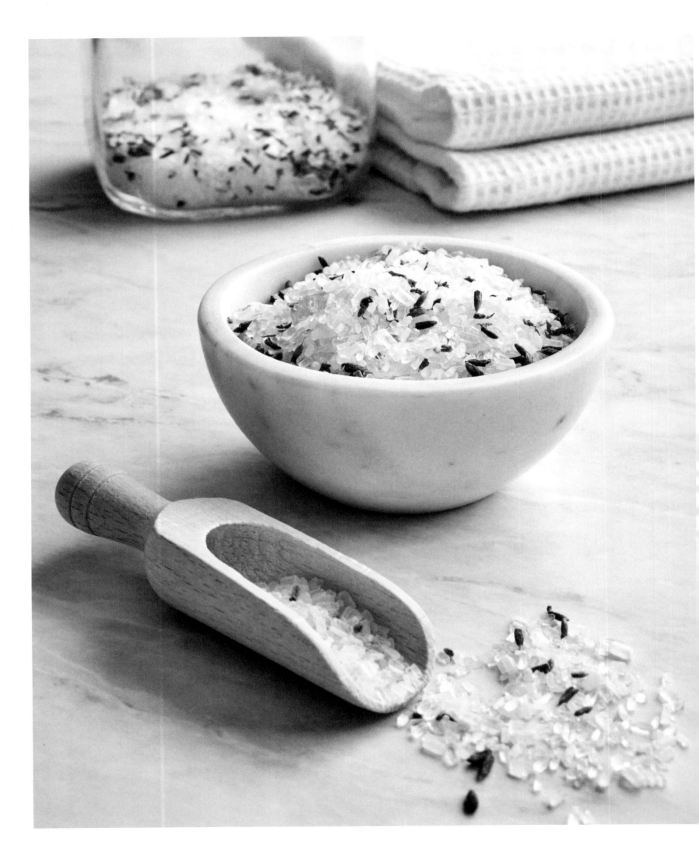

AROMATHERAPEUTIC BATH SALTS

Bath time will be even more relaxing with these CBD- and essential oil–infused bath salts. Epsom salts soothe sore muscles and essential oils relieve tension. Use as much or as little as you need—one or two scoops should be enough for the relief you are seeking.

TIME: 5 MINUTES	MAKES: 3 CUPS (600G)	CONTAINER: STERILE GLASS JAR

3 cups (600g) all-natural, rough-cut Epsom salts

2 tsp (10ml) or less CBD oil

20 drops pine or spruce essential oil

15 drops melissa (lemon balm) essential oil

10 drops rosemary essential oil

2 tbsp (8g) dried lavender flowers

1. Place the Epsom salts in a dry, sterile glass jar. Stirring thoroughly after each addition, add the desired amount of CBD oil along with the essential oil drops of pine or spruce, melissa, and rosemary one at a time to evenly distribute the oils throughout the Epsom salts. Fold the lavender flowers into the salts until evenly distributed.

2. Store in a glass container with a tightly closed lid. A silicone-based moisture absorbing packet kept inside of the jar with the bath salts is suggested for keeping this fresh. Use within 3 months for best results.

TO USE:

Add the bath salts to an empty tub and begin filling with hot water. After the tub has reached ¼ full, and all bath salts have melted, begin adjusting the water temperature to your liking, and finish filling the tub.

FOLK HEALER RUB

There are many folk healing traditions throughout the world that include cannabis and hemp. This modern CBD-infused recipe is an interpretation of tincture-based folk medicine rubs and is meant for external use to treat sore muscles and joints.

TIME: 2–4 WEEKS	MAKES: 16OZ (480ML)	CONTAINER: STERILE GLASS BOTTLE OR JAR

16oz (480ml) 150-proof or higher clear alcohol (tequila, rum, or grain spirits)
1 bunch of fresh spearmint
1 bunch of fresh rosemary
1 bunch of fresh thyme (lemon thyme is preferable if available)
½ cup (60g) fresh or dried juniper berries
2 tsp (10ml) or less CBD oil

1. In a glass jar with a lid, layer the spearmint, rosemary, thyme, and juniper berries in even amounts. Add the alcohol and press down to allow for about ½ inch of the alcohol to cover all of the herbs.

2. Close the lid tightly and place in a cool, dark cabinet. Allow the herbs to steep in the alcohol for up to 4 weeks. Shake once a week.

3. Decant and strain the alcohol from the herbs into a lidded glass jar or bottle for storage. Discard the herbs. Add the CBD oil and shake to infuse it into the alcohol. Use within 6 months for best results.

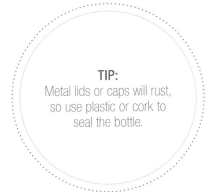

TIP:
Metal lids or caps will rust, so use plastic or cork to seal the bottle.

TO USE:
Pour a small amount into your hand and massage into sore muscles or joints. Keep tightly closed when not in use. Do not apply to broken or irritated skin, and keep away from heat and open flames.

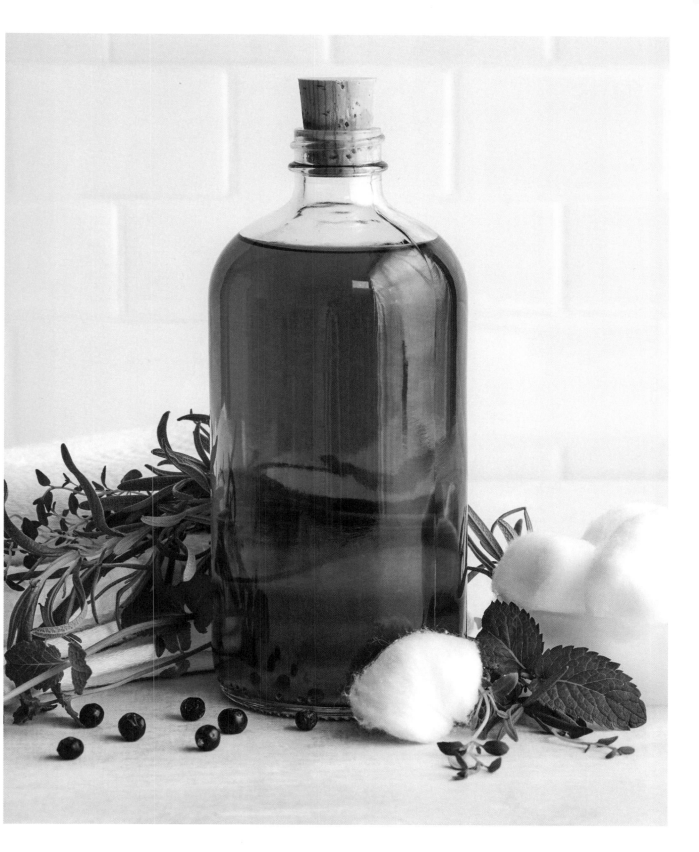

INDEX

About the Author

Dr. Rachna Patel is an internationally recognized expert in the field of medical cannabis. Through her courses and consultations, she offers a clear understanding of what to expect when using CBD products, while also dispelling fears people may have about the treatment and putting their minds at ease. She has helped people from many countries manage a wide range of medical conditions including anxiety, chronic pain, insomnia, and more.

Dr. Patel completed her undergraduate studies at Northwestern University (IL) and earned her medical degree from Touro University (CA). While training in emergency medicine, she witnessed the shortcomings of conventional medicines in relieving pain and ventured into the field of medical cannabis instead. Eventually, she started her own practice to offer quality care that's otherwise not available in the field of medical cannabis.

Dr. Patel's knowledge of CBD has made her an asset in the specialty. She has been interviewed on over 200 podcasts, has taken the stage worldwide to spread awareness, has been featured in articles for Lifehacker and mindbodygreen, and has appeared on major news networks.

Connect with her and find helpful articles, online programs, and more at DrRachnaPatel.com.

Acknowledgments

There's not enough space in this book to express my wholehearted gratitude to each and every person who supported me to this end. Some have been there throughout. Others, I serendipitously met along the way. Regardless, each and every one of you touched my life in a way that propelled the conviction to change the lives of millions. And here we are today. Thank you.

About the Recipes

All recipes were developed by **Sandra Hinchliffe,** a home herbalist, allergy chef, and author based in Del Norte County, California. She is the founder of posyandkettle.com, where she shares recipes and more. Her books include *The Cannabis Spa at Home* and *High Tea.*